# Biochemical Parameters and the Nutritional Status of Children

# Biochemical Parameters and the Nutritional Status of Children

## Novel Tools for Assessment

**Anil Gupta, PhD**
Dean of Research
Desh Bhagat University
and
Professor and Head
Department of Physiology and Biochemistry
Desh Bhagat Dental College and Hospital
Mandi Gobindgarh
Punjab, India

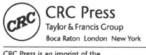

**CRC Press**
Taylor & Francis Group
Boca Raton London New York

CRC Press is an imprint of the
Taylor & Francis Group, an **informa** business

First edition published 2020
by CRC Press
6000 Broken Sound Parkway NW, Suite 300, Boca Raton, FL 33487-2742

and by CRC Press
2 Park Square, Milton Park, Abingdon, Oxon, OX14 4RN

First issued in paperback 2022

**Visit the Taylor & Francis Web site at**
http://www.taylorandfrancis.com

**and the CRC Press Web site at**
http://www.crcpress.com

Library of Congress Cataloging-in-Publication Data
Names: Gupta, Anil (Child nutrition scientist), author.
Title: Biochemical parameters and the nutritional status of children:
novel tools for assessment / by Anil Gupta.
Description: First edition. | Boca Raton: CRC Press, 2020. |
Includes bibliographical references and index. |
Summary: "Biochemical parameters represent better, precise, and objective tools toward
the assessment of nutritional status of children in comparison to anthropometric,
clinical, and dietary methods. They constitute laboratory tests to estimate the
concentration of circulating nutrients in the body fluids" – Provided by publisher.
Identifiers: LCCN 2020006248 (print) | LCCN 2020006249 (ebook) |
ISBN 9780367419813 (hardback) | ISBN 9780367419820 (ebook)
Subjects: MESH: Nutritional Status | Child | Child Nutrition
Disorders–diagnosis | Clinical Laboratory Techniques
Classification: LCC RJ206 (print) | LCC RJ206 (ebook) |
NLM WS 130 | DDC 362.1963/9–dc23
LC record available at https://lccn.loc.gov/2020006248
LC ebook record available at https://lccn.loc.gov/2020006249

ISBN: 978-0-367-49857-3 (pbk)
ISBN: 978-0-367-41981-3 (hbk)
ISBN: 978-0-367-41982-0 (ebk)

DOI: 10.1201/9780367419820

TypesetinMinion
by Newgen Publishing UK

I dedicate my book to the Almighty,
SHRI SHIRDI SAI BABA

# Contents

# Preface

B IOCHEMICAL PARAMETERS REPRESENT superior, precise, and objective tools toward the assessment of nutritional status of children in comparison to anthropometric, clinical, and dietary methods. Biochemical parameters estimate the nutrients in the body through laboratory methods and should be interpreted in conformity with the other methods of assessment of the nutritional status of children. Biochemical parameters are suggestive of acute or subclinical conditions when the other methods of nutritional assessment fail to interpret the condition.

These parameters constitute laboratory tests to estimate the concentration of circulating nutrients in body fluids, while the other tests explore the concentration of enzymes in the body tissues, representing the metabolic changes. Biochemical parameters exhibit substantial variability in their reproducibility. Moreover, these parameters are novel tools in the hands of clinicians for the screening of the nutritional status of children.

This book provides useful information about the role of biochemical parameters in assessing the nutritional status of children.

# Acknowledgments

THE ALMIGHTY, SHRI SHIRDI SAI BABA, bestows upon me the knowledge and perseverance for preparing the book.

My father, Sh. Ved Parkash Gupta, always inspires me to achieve high goals. I am highly indebted to my parents for inspiring me toward academics since my school days.

I am thankful to my wife, Dr. Deepali Gupta, for her support in data collection, designing the draft, and writing the manuscript.

I am thankful to my daughter, Deeksha Gupta, MBBS student for her assistance in compiling the manuscript.

I owe my gratitude to Dr. Renu Upadhyay for focusing my attention toward the Taylor & Francis publication team with my proposal. I am sincerely grateful to Dr. Shivangi Pramanik for initiating and pursuing efforts for the publication of this book.

I express my thanks to Himani Dwivedi and the team of CRC Press/Taylor & Francis for their support, cooperation, and gentle attitude in fulfilling my dream.

# About the Author

**Anil Gupta, PhD,** is currently serving as Dean of Research at Desh Bhagat University and Professor and Head in the Department of Physiology and Biochemistry at Desh Bhagat Dental College and Hospital, Mandi Gobindgarh in Punjab, India.

He graduated in biosciences from Punjab University in 1989. He obtained his bachelor's in dental surgery from the University of Poona in 1984. Later, he completed his master's in biochemistry in 2009 and his PhD in biochemistry in 2012 from SJJT University, Rajasthan.

He is persistently pursuing postdoctoral research at Srinivas University in Mangaluru in Karnataka, India. His postdoctoral research is related to the nutritional status of children between two years to under five years of age. He has presented research papers in reputed universities such as Thaper University, Patiala; Birla Institute of Technology and Sciences, Pilani; Punjabi University, Patiala; M.D. University, Rohtak; and Arya P.G. College under Kurukshetra University.

He has more than 30 research papers to his credit and has been accepted and published in high-impact, peer-reviewed, and indexed journals. During his academic career, he has been awarded merit certificates, merit scholarships, and gold and silver medals.

He has more than 11 years of teaching experience, seven years of postdoctoral experience, and five years of PhD supervisor experience; as well as more than 23 years of clinical experience. He is a guide to PhD scholars in universities. He supervises research scholars in distinctive fields, including heavy metals contamination of water, quality analysis of drinking water, and predisposition of blood groups to diabetes mellitus and dyslipidemia. He serves as adjunct faculty to teach research methodology to research scholars in universities.

Additionally, he serves as a reviewer and member of editorial boards of national and international journals. His research interests are focused on human physiology (oral cavity, saliva, deglutition), nutrition, and associated pathophysiology. He is an international author, whose work includes titles such as *Nutritional Anemia in Preschool Children, Comprehensive Biochemistry for Dentistry: A Textbook for Dental Students* (comprising a separate chapter on dental biochemistry covering salivary composition, functions, enamel, dentine), and *Geophagia: History, Epidemiology and Etiology.*

# CHAPTER 1

# Concept of Nutrition

## THE MEANING OF NUTRITION

Nutrition is the sum of physiological activities comprising intake of food, its digestion, absorption, assimilation, and egestion of undigested foodstuff from the alimentary canal. Nutrition is the science dealing with the intake of food and its effect on the growth and development of the human body (Cambridge Dictionary 2019). The word *nutrition* is taken from the Latin "nutritio" that signifies, "nurture" or "feeding."

The science of nutrition deals with the interaction of nutrients with the body tissues and studies how the nutrients affect the living tissues of the body and what the body does to the nutrients (U.S. National Library of Medicine 2019; Whitney and Rolfes 2013).

According to the World Health Organization (WHO 2019), the living body needs energy to perform mental and physical activities. The energy need of the body is fulfilled through the intake of nutrients. A balanced diet is necessary for maintenance of health, whereas inadequate nutrition results in malnutrition, repeated infections, and delayed growth and development (WHO 2019).

According to the U.S. National Library of Medicine (USNLM 1998), the science of nutrition deals with every phase of interaction between food and body tissues. The USNLM (1998) explains the term *clinical nutrition* and defines it as the branch of the science of nutrition that studies the prevention, diagnosis, and treatment of various nutritional and metabolic diseases either in acute or chronic forms due to either deficiency or excess of calories and nutrients.

## HISTORY OF HUMAN NUTRITION

### Ancient Concept of Nutrition

The first dietary suggestion that was recorded in human civilization probably dates from around 2500 BCE; in the form of a carving in Babylonian stone, and recommended abstaining from onions for three days so as to heal internal pain. This age-old advice was reported by Payne-Palacio and Canter (2014), who also discuss the 1500 BCE description of scurvy found in the Ebers Papyrus.

Ayurveda—a traditional medicinal system that originated around 3,000 to 4,000 years ago in the Indian subcontinent—provides exhaustive narrations about food, health, and diseases. Ahara (nutrition) in Ayurveda is the cornerstone of body health and disease. Ahara is mentioned as one of the three prime concepts of life, the other two being sleep and controlled sexual life. In around 600 BCE in the Sanskrit text *Taittiriya Upanishad*, Ahara (nutrition) had been described as *Brahma* (the creator of universe) owing to its prime essentiality in sustaining life. The energy for growth and development for living organisms is derived from food/Ahara (Nathani 2014).

Another Sanskrit text from around 600 BCE, the *Sushruta Samhita*, mentioned elaborately the value of Ahara and dependency of human life on the correct Ahara (food) and Vihara (lifestyle) (Shastri 2003).

According to Gratzer (2005), a British biophysical chemist, the science of nutrition emerged around 600 BCE. It was around this time that foods were classified in India, China, Persia, and Malaysia. Foods such as meat, ginger, blood, and spices were kept in the category of hot foods, while food items like green vegetables were mentioned as cold food by the author (Gratzer 2005).

According to Gratzer (2005), Ho, a physician in China around 600 BCE, mentioned that deficiency of elements like water, wood, fire, metal, and earth in the body of individuals was responsible for the onset of diseases.

Furthermore, Gratzer (2005) reports the written account of a Greek, Alcmaeon of Croton, around 600 BCE, in Italy. Alcmaeon mentions the importance of equilibrium between the intake of food and excretion of undigested matter from the body, which was important in deciding the health of a person and onset of a disease like obesity or wasting.

According to authors Gratzer (2005) and Smith (2004), in around 400 BCE Hippocrates mentioned that food should be selected judiciously so that it may become medicine for the person, and that medicine ought to become food so as to normalize the pathological state of the person. Hippocrates advocated the prudent use of food and performing sufficient physical exercise to help prevent the onset of disease and obesity.

## Medieval Concept of Nutrition

Galen was a famous physician of the gladiators in the Roman Empire, and also treated Marcus Aurelius, the emperor in Rome in around 130–200 CE (Gratzer 2005). Regarding nutrition, Galen mentioned the concept of "humors of body" of Hippocrates— black bile, yellow bile, phlegm, and blood, pertaining to four temperaments of individuals. These "humors" described the constitution of the human body and provided the basis for the medicinal system in Ancient Rome and Greece.

Galen described the concept of *pneuma*, a Greek word meaning soul or breath, which was considered the essence of life that pervaded in the body organs (Gratzer 2005).

Around 1500, Paracelsus and Leonardo da Vinci severely criticized the work of Galen (Gratzer 2005). British Navy physician James Lind was the first person who performed scientific work on nutrition. It was found that sailors who were at sea for prolonged periods suffered from a fatal disorder involving swollen gums, known as scurvy. It was James Lind who discovered that lime juice could cure patients from scurvy (Willet and Skerrett 2005). According to Gratzer (2005), it was Antoine Lavoisier in around 1770 who described metabolism. He discovered that oxidation of foodstuff could generate energy. Antoine Lavoisier, along with his assistant Armand Seguin, estimated the respiratory output of carbonic acid in humans at rest and while lifting weights (Kenneth 2003; Seguin and Lavoisier 1789).

In 1816, French physiologist and surgeon François Magendie conducted his famous experiments on dogs. He used a nutritious food (sugar) to feed dogs. Initially, the first dog ate well for a period of two weeks and was healthy. Thereafter, a corneal ulcer developed in the dog and it lost weight (Magendie 1816; Kenneth 2003). It died after a month. The feeding experiment was repeated with a second dog, by providing a diet rich in olive oil, butter, or gum. The corneal ulcer was not observed in the dog that was fed olive oil, otherwise the dogs fell ill and died (Magendie 1816; Kenneth 2003).

Magendie demonstrated that a protein-deficient diet containing carbohydrates, lipids, and water could not save the dogs from starvation, while a diet enriched with proteins could prevent starvation and provide all the nutritional needs of the dog. The experiment proved the health benefits of proteins in the food for living organisms (Magendie 1816; Kenneth 2003).

According to Ahrens (1977), in 1827, it was English chemist William Prout who was the first person to propose the elements as carbohydrates, fat, and protein that are constituents of food.

In 1860, the French physiologist Claude Bernard demonstrated the glycogenic role of the liver that proved vital for the discovery of diabetes mellitus (Young 1957).

In the 1880s, Takaki Kanehiro (who served in the Imperial Japanese Navy as a physician) reported that some Japanese sailors developed beriberi disease. It was observed by Takaki that the sailors consumed white rice only as food and he concluded the disease to be associated with the intake of white rice. He confirmed that beriberi was unheard of among British sailors and naval officers in Japan due to their diet containing meat and vegetables (Bay 2012; Low 2005). However, physicians from Tokyo Imperial University declared beriberi as an infectious disease (Bay 2012; Low 2005).

## THE MODERN CONCEPT OF NUTRITION

In the early years of the twentieth century, Carl von Voit was a German physiologist and pioneer in modern dietetics. He performed substantive work in estimation of the constituents of excreted urea under varying food intake conditions. He concluded that the quantity of nitrogenous substances in excreted urea was independent of the intake of nitrogenous dietary components, although it depends on the nutritional status of the person (Kafatos and Hatzis 2008). It is attributed to the varying needs of nitrogen to body tissues under different conditions as pregnancy, lactation, and diseases (Kafatos and Hatzis 2008).

Tryptophan is an essential amino acid. Its necessity for the normal growth and development of organisms was demonstrated by Willcock and Hopkins in 1906 (Peters 1991). Later in 1914, Osborne and Mendel described the essentiality of tryptophan for growth in mice and rats. Moreover, in 1957, Rose announced that tryptophan is the essential amino acid that is to be supplemented with diet for sustaining normal growth of individuals (Peters 1991).

In 1912, the English biochemist Sir Frederick Gowland Hopkins performed a series of feeding experiments on rats. He fed rats a diet containing an adequate quantity of essential nutrients such as proteins, fats, carbohydrates, and minerals, but the diet could not support the growth of rats. He concluded that some trace elements were missing from the diet that were vital for the growth and weight gain of animals and he named them as "essential food factors," which were the vitamins (Hopkins 1912).

## PHASE OF VITAMINS

In 1912, Casimir Funk proposed that a complex chemical substance in unpolished rice could protect chickens from beriberi disease and he named it *anti-beriberi factor* and coined the term "vitamine" describing the complex as important and vital "amine" for the normal growth and development of the body. It was assumed by Funk that these vital substances were necessary for growth and for prevention of diseases. Later in 1926, the complex chemical substance that was isolated from unpolished rice was found to be thiamine (vitamin B1) (Eijkman 1929).

In 1913, Elmer McCollum discovered vitamin A and vitamin B. In 1919, Sir Edward Mellanby correlated the deficiency of vitamin A with rickets. He worked on cod liver oil and successfully treated rickets in dogs. Later in 1922, McCollum destroyed the vitamin A in the cod liver oil and fed the sick dogs this modified cod liver oil, and it still cured the dogs from rickets. McCollum concluded the presence of a substance in cod liver oil that could cure rickets that was different from vitamin A, and which was named vitamin D (Wolf 2004; Elena 2006; McClean and Budy 1964).

In 1925, Edwin B. Hart demonstrated that minute quantity of copper could stimulate iron absorption from the gastrointestinal tract (GIT). In 1928, Adolf Windaus was awarded the Nobel Prize in chemistry for his work on chemical structure of sterols and their link with vitamins (Windaus 1928). The sterols were vitamin D.

Albert Szent-Györgyi isolated ascorbic acid in 1928. Later in 1932, he commented on the role of ascorbic acid in the prophylaxis of scurvy. In 1937, he was awarded the Nobel Prize for synthesizing ascorbic acid.

In 1930, American nutritionist and biochemist William Cumming Rose's work at Illinois was concentrated upon the metabolism of amino acids. His work documented the role of essential amino acids in growth. He discovered the amino acid threonine and published his work in 1949 as "Amino Acid Requirements of Man."

Erhard Fernholz, a German chemist who worked on bile acids and sterols, described the chemical structure of vitamin E in 1938 (Evans et al. 1936).

In 1940, nutritional principles were forwarded by British nutritionist Elsie Widdowson. She supervised the government-mandated program of supplementation of vitamins to food and also undertook the project of rationing in the UK during World War II. Under this project, she led the program of the addition of calcium to bread. In 1942, Elsie Widdowson documented that health could be maintained by intake of a limited amount of food with the addition of calcium supplements. Her work was supported by the Minister of Food, Lord Woolton (Elliot 2007).

In 1941, the National Research Council provided the first Recommended Dietary Allowances (RDAs). In 1992, the United States Department of Agriculture provided the concept of the Food Guide Pyramid that was replaced in 2005 by MyPyramid, which was provided by the USDA Center for Nutrition Policy and Promotion. The symbol of MyPyramid shows an individual stepping up on stairs depicting physical activity. Further, the vertical lines in MyPyramid show mixing of food groups and allocation of the amounts of food (USDA 2019; USDHHS 2005a,b).

In 2011, MyPyramid was further replaced by MyPlate, which is the working nutrition program provided by the USDA Center for Nutrition Policy and Promotion. MyPlate comprises a colored circle that depicts a plate, which is divided into four groups— vegetables, fruits, proteins, and grains. The plate also has a small circle of dairy, thus describing the overall five food groups for health (USDA 2019).

- Macronutrients for health

  - Proteins

  - Carbohydrates

  - Lipids

  - Fibers

  - Essential fatty acids

## NUTRIENTS

A nutrient is a chemical substance that is derived from food and is essential for normal growth, development, and repair of tissues of the body.

Nutrients are broadly classified into two groups—macronutrients and micronutrients. The former group of nutrients is required by the body in large quantities and either produces energy in body tissues or is incorporated into tissues for repair and regeneration (except dietary fibers and water), while the latter group of nutrients is taken in small amounts that serve as coenzymes and cofactors in biochemical reactions of the body. The macronutrients include proteins, carbohydrates, water, and lipids, while the micronutrients are vitamins and minerals (Center for Food Safety 2019).

## CARBOHYDRATES

Carbohydrates constitute an essential component of human food. These are necessary to meet the energy requirement of a healthy person who needs nearly 2,800 calories daily. Daily intake of carbohydrates should be adjusted so that around 60% of the total calories is derived from the carbohydrates. The caloric value of carbohydrates is around 4 kcal per gram. Accordingly, a healthy individual must consume around 450 grams of carbohydrates as macronutrients daily to meet the required proportion of calories. Moreover, carbohydrates constitute the main building block of the daily dietary demand in the financially poorer sections of society. About 90% of the calories consumed by people of low socioeconomic status are derived from carbohydrates.

Dietary carbohydrates can be grouped as monosaccharides, disaccharides, and polysaccharides. The monosaccharides are the simplest sugars. The monosaccharides are the major structural carbohydrates in wheat, rice, maize, oats, and other cereals. Disaccharides and polysaccharides contain two and more than two monosaccharide units.

Monosaccharides as hexoses—namely fructose, glucose, galactose, and mannose—represent the major source of energy for the body, whereas, pentoses—namely ribose and deoxyribose—are involved in the synthesis of nucleic acids, as pentoses have poor nutritional and caloric values. Hexoses constitute a major proportion of the daily diet. Disaccharides, such as sucrose, maltose, and lactose, and polysaccharides like starch and glycogen are macromolecules and are hydrolyzed in the lumen of alimentary canal into monosaccharides.

Carbohydrates have a direct influence on the metabolism of lipids and proteins. Inadequate intake of carbohydrates invariably disturbs the metabolism of lipids. The tissue lipase is activated. The mobilization of fats from the adipose tissues is increased. There is exaggerated lipolysis at tissue level leading to a rise in the concentration of free fatty acids in the blood circulation. As a consequence, the rate of ketogenesis is enhanced, resulting in a rise in plasma keto bodies (ketonemia) and excretion of keto bodies in urine (ketonuria). These are features of ketosis resulting from the absence of adequate dietary carbohydrates in an individual's daily diet and can lead to disease, such as uncontrolled diabetes mellitus.

Adequate intake of carbohydrates has a protein sparing effect (obtaining energy from macronutrients other than proteins). The carbohydrates and fats in a diet provide energy to body tissues so that the catabolism of tissue proteins is spared for production of energy. Simultaneously, the dietary carbohydrates also provide non-essential amino acids. The intermediate metabolites of carbohydrate metabolism like glycolysis and the TCA cycle provide pyruvate, oxaloacetate, and alpha ketoglutarate, which enter into the transamination process and are converted into non-essential amino acids like alanine, aspartate, and glutamate.

Carbohydrates have an influence on nitrogen excretion from the body. A carbohydrate-restricted diet leads to an increase in nitrogen excretion, while the calorie requirement of the person is fulfilled through proportional increase (iso-caloric) in the intake of fat. The consumption of carbohydrates decreases the excretion of nitrogen, while the intake of fats has no effect on nitrogen excretion.

Carbohydrates can directly or indirectly influence the predisposing factors of diseases or the pathogenesis of diseases. The prevalence of obesity has increased alarmingly worldwide in developed as well as developing countries. This has a substantive negative impact on the health of persons, predisposing them to diabetes mellitus, coronary artery disease, hypertension, and atherosclerosis. Genetic factors, a sedentary lifestyle, and environmental factors also contribute to the onset of obesity (FAO 2019).

There is ambiguity regarding the involvement of a carbohydrate-rich diet in the pathogenesis of obesity. Solid-form carbohydrates in a diet induce a sense of satiety and, in the long term, reduce the prevalence of obesity; contrarily, liquid-form carbohydrates, like sweetened beverages, are unable to produce satiety and their repeated intake can lead to gain in body weight and thus obesity. Moreover, dietary fibers are cellulose-rich components of food that have no caloric value but roughage value. These are prominently found in vegetables, fruits, and whole-grain cereals that are linked significantly with weight management and reduction of obesity (Gaesser 2007).

Dietary fibers from legumes, cereals, vegetables, and fruits as well as carbohydrates with a low glycemic index are beneficial in controlling hyperglycemia and prevention of non-insulin-dependent diabetes mellitus. Changes in culture, dietary habits, and lifestyle have contributed substantially to the cause of diabetes mellitus. Dietary carbohydrates have not been directly implicated in the cause of diabetes mellitus (FAO 2019).

Non-starch polysaccharides occurring in natural foods like vegetables, fruits, and whole grains are enriched with antioxidants. Their intake helps to reduce the level of pro-oxidants in body and minimize the risk for oxidative stress. These carbohydrates have a preventive role in the cause of coronary artery disease. Carbohydrates like beta-glucans have an important role in lowering the serum cholesterol level. These are beneficial in the management of atherosclerosis and hypercholesterolemia, which are significant causal factors in the onset of coronary artery disease (FAO 2019).

Foods containing sugars or starch may be easily broken down by α-amylase and bacteria in the mouth. This alters the pH of saliva and can produce acid which increases the risk of dental caries. Moreover, the type of carbohydrates, frequency of intake, oral hygiene, pH of saliva, salivary flow, and fluoride application have independent and interrelated effects on the production of acids and progression of dental caries (FAO 2019).

## DIETARY FIBERS

Dietary fibers are the plant-obtained food substances that are not digested in the human alimentary canal. The term "dietary fiber" was coined by Hipsley in 1953 (Hipsley 1953).

According to the British Nutrition Foundation (2018), dietary fibers constitute a group of complex organic food substances derived from plants, which are resistant to the digestive juices in the alimentary canal of humans.

Dietary fibers include non-starch polysaccharides like cellulose, limit dextrins, inulins, chitins, lignins, beta-glucans, pectins, and oligosaccharides. Dietary fibers are thought to be indigestible in the gut of humans and have no calorific value. However, they do have roughage value. Additionally, some dietary fibers are soluble in water and are fermented in the colon by the colonic bacteria and produce gases and short-chain fatty acids.

Trowell (1972) broadened the scope of dietary fibers as polysaccharides that are resistant to digestion in the human gut and include substances like cellulose, gum, mucilage, pectins, and oligosaccharides that are mostly saccharides of plant storage.

In 1998, the president of the American Association of Cereal Chemists (AACC) formed a scientific committee to review the definition of dietary fibers. According to the AACC (1998, 2001) dietary fibers are defined as the edible parts of plants or analogous carbohydrates that are resistant to digestion and absorption in the human small intestine with complete or partial fermentation in the large intestine.

The Institute of Medicine (2001) defines dietary fibers as non-digestible carbohydrates and lignins (phenolic compounds that are attached covalently to polysaccharides), which are the intrinsic parts of the plants and remain intact inside plants. Dietary fibers include parts of the plant food that have intact cells and plant matrix. They also contain macronutrients like proteins, carbohydrates, and lipids. Bran consists of dietary fibers, proteins, and starch and it is the outermost layer of wheat kernel that has a hard consistency.

The Institute of Medicine (2001) further defined "added fibers" as the non-digestible carbohydrates that are extracted from natural plant foods and have physiological benefits to humans. Added fibers include the ones that are prepared commercially or the extracted oligosaccharides that are found in nature (Institute of Medicine 2001). The Institute of Medicine (2001) also introduced the new term "total fibers" as the sum total of dietary fibers and added fibers.

Dietary fibers are also classified into two categories—soluble fibers and insoluble fibers. The former group of fibers is soluble in water. Soluble fibers are subjected to fermentation by colonic bacteria in the colon of humans. There is formation of gases and short chain fatty acids. Soluble fibers are mucilaginous and viscous and delay the gastric emptying. Examples of soluble fibers include fructans, pectins, inulin, alginic acid, raffinose, lactulose, and xylose.

The latter group of fibers is insoluble in water. Insoluble fibers are not digested in the lumen of the alimentary canal of humans. These fibers have no nutritional or caloric value, and add bulk to the large intestine. These fibers absorb water in the lumen of the large intestine and increase the volume of stools. These fibers have roughage value and promote peristaltic movements, helping in the evacuation of bowels and relieving constipation. Examples of insoluble fibers include cellulose, hemicellulose, chitin, lignin, and xanthan gum.

Dietary fibers have a bulking effect and roughage value. These fibers increase the bulk of stools that are easier to evacuate.

A fiber-rich diet decreases the chances of colorectal cancer. Kunzmann et al. (2005) selected participants from a Prostate, Lung, Colorectal, and Ovarian Cancer Screening Trial. The authors reported that the consumption of maximum dietary fibers in a routine diet have a profound suppressing effect over the incidence of distal colon cancer and colorectal adenoma. They further commented that the fibers should be derived from vegetables, cereals, and fruits (Kunzmann et al. 2005).

Sengupta et al. (2006) and Lipkin et al. (1999) posited the possible mechanism of intake of fibers and reduction in the chances of colorectal cancer. It was presumed that bacteria ferment the fibers in the colon and produce short-chain fatty acids that could have anti-carcinogenic effect on the body tissues. Further, the intake of fibers could dilute the effective concentration of carcinogens in the colon.

The soluble dietary fiber in flaxseed, oats, and wheat kernel bran could help decrease the serum cholesterol level. These fibers are helpful in hypercholesterolemia and could play a role in the prophylaxis of coronary artery disease.

Gunness and Gidley (2010) mentioned that multiple studies proved a direct and positive relation between the intake of foods rich in soluble dietary fibers like psyllium, guar gum, beta-glucan, and pectin and the reduction in the incidence of coronary artery disease. The authors posited that the plausible mechanism is the enhanced excretion of bile salts from the lumen of the small intestine through reduced reabsorption of bile salts in the small intestine by the soluble dietary fibers. Additionally, the fibers induce a lower rate of absorption of sugars from the mucosa of the small intestine and thus sustain a lower glycemic response (Gunness and Gidley 2010). This reduces the synthesis of cholesterol in the liver through decreased activation of insulin.

Soluble dietary fibers have benefits in the control of type 2 diabetes mellitus. The soluble dietary fibers decrease the digestion of carbohydrates in the alimentary canal and subsequently reduce the rate of absorption of sugars from intestinal mucosa. Therefore, the fibers help in the control of post-prandial hyperglycemia. These fibers also provide a sense of satiety and reduce the intake of food that ensures a decrease in body weight (American Diabetes Association 2013; Post et al. 2012).

## PROTEINS

Proteins are an essential constituent of the routine diet of humans. These form nearly 12 kg dry weight of the human body in an adult individual of 70 kg. Proteins in the human body are comprised of a total of 20 amino acids. In adults, eight amino acids are considered essential amino acids (threonine, tryptophan, phenyl alanine, valine, methionine, isoleucine, leucine, and lysine), as these are supplemented with diet and are not synthesized by body tissues. In children, the amino acids arginine and histidine, along with the eight earlier essential amino acids, are considered as conditionally essential amino acids, as children are unable to synthesize adequate arginine and histidine amino acids in their body to meet the daily requirement of these amino acids. The remaining ten amino acids are considered as non-essential amino acids, as these are synthesized by the body tissues.

Proteins serve as structural and functional components of the human body and are necessary for synthesis and repair of body tissues. Proteins intensively influence the growth and development of body tissues. The caloric value of 1 g of protein is nearly 4 kcal.

An adult healthy person should consume nearly 0.8 g of protein per kilogram of body weight daily. The total protein intake per day is around 560 g for an adult male with 70 kg body weight. The RDA of proteins in physiological conditions like pregnancy and lactation rises. The children in formative years (1–5 years) require around 30–40 g protein per day. The protein requirement in aged individuals, convalescents, and during chronic disease, such as cirrhosis and renal failure, increases.

The proteins from the food enter the alimentary canal and are digested by the action of proteolytic enzymes into constituent amino acids. These are absorbed through the mucosa of the small intestine and enter blood circulation. The free amino acids reach the liver via the hepatic portal vein. The amino acids enter the amino acid pool of the body and are also utilized for synthesis and repair of body tissues. Conversely, tissue proteins are decomposed to release amino acids that enrich the amino acid pool. Amino acids in the body are in a dynamic state.

The surplus amino acids are in the phase of catabolism. These are subjected to a biochemical process of transamination wherein the surplus amino acid is converted into alpha keto acid that enters the TCA cycle and is utilized for production of energy. The excess amino acid also undergoes deamination, through which it is converted into alpha keto acid with the release of ammonia. It is transported to the liver where it is converted into urea that enters blood circulation and is excreted by kidneys.

The proteins are derived from the plant- and animal-based sources in the diet. The quality of protein from animal sources is considered better in comparison to proteins that are obtained from plant foods. The quality of proteins is based on the amino acids present in that protein. The sequence of amino acids in animal proteins is comparable to that of proteins in human body tissues, while the opposite is true about the plant proteins.

The presence of all the essential amino acids in the protein makes it a complete protein, while the absence of one or more essential amino acid yields an incomplete protein.

The proteins from animal sources are complete proteins, which provide all the essential amino acids. Examples include proteins from meat, fish, eggs, and cheese. Plant-based proteins are incomplete proteins. The combination of foods has a complementary effect on the proteins. Thus, the intake of cereal and pulses in a diet complement the one incomplete protein with another and the mixed food yields complete essential amino acids to individuals. Examples of plant proteins can be soya proteins, cereals, pulses, and nuts.

The quality of the protein is also important and depends on the amino acids that are present. Proteins from animal sources have a higher biological value than proteins from plant sources. This is because the pattern of amino acids in animal cells is comparable to the pattern in human cells. Plant foods may have very different patterns of amino acids compared to animal proteins, and, in the past, this difference has led to a concept of first-class and second-class proteins, for animal and plant foods, respectively. However, diets are typically varied and rarely made up of single foods. A combination of plant proteins tends to have a complementary effect, boosting their overall biological value.

## LIPIDS

Triglycerides, cholesterol, and phospholipids constitute around 95% of the total lipids in a routine diet for a healthy person. Lipids are the chief energy-producing macromolecules in the body. An adult and healthy person of 70 kg requires around 2,800 calories daily for light work. It is advisable that nearly 20% to 35% of the total calories per day must be derived from lipids in the diet.

The caloric value of dietary lipids is 9 kcal per gram of lipids. It is recommended that an adult individual must take nearly 60–90 g of fats daily in their diet. Additionally, the calorie intake from the saturated fatty acids and trans-fatty acids must be reduced to 10% and 0–2% of total calories per day, respectively.

Dietary lipids are helpful in the transport of fat-soluble vitamins in the body. The lipids serve as carriers of vitamins like A, D, E, and K along with beta-carotene. These vitamins are soluble in fats and are distributed from one organ to another.

Dietary lipids have a satiety effect in humans. The lipids control the intake of food through multiple mechanisms. Dietary fats regulate the secretion of ghrelin and leptin, which are appetite hormones. These hormones in turn control the appetite and induce a sense of satiety. Lipids decrease gastric emptying, which provides a sense of fullness and reduces the intake of food, helping in weight loss (Samra 2010).

The dietary lipids should have a sufficient quantity of polyunsaturated fatty acids (PUFAs). There should be a minimum amount of

PUFAs in the diet so that around 1% of the total calories are derived from PUFAs in adults (NIH 2019). PUFAs are found in high concentration in the biomembranes in humans. Polyunsaturated fatty acids constitute the substrate for the action of enzymes in the synthesis of prostaglandins and leukotrienes. The arachidonic acid from the plasma membrane of cells produces the prostaglandin through action of cyclooxygenase enzyme, while the enzyme lipoxygenase catalyzes the synthesis of leukotrienes from arachidonic acid in the leukocytes (Ricciotti and FitzGerald 2011).

Docosahexaenoic acid (DHA) is the polyenoic acid that is abundantly found in the cell membranes of cones and rods in the retina. DHA is synthesized from linolenic acid that is taken in the diet. DHA is essential for the functioning of photoreceptor cells and both DHA and linolenic acid are vital for normal vision (Calder 2016).

Trans-fatty acids possess one or more double-bonds that are in the trans configuration instead of the cis configuration. The trans-fats are directly associated with coronary artery disease, disorder of vision, breast cancer, preeclampsia, obesity, and diabetes mellitus in humans. Trans-fatty acids in diet have a profound negative impact on the concentration of high-density lipoproteins, while they increase the concentration of low-density lipoproteins and level of insulin.

The dietary lipids are comprised of saturated fatty acids, mono-unsaturated, and polyunsaturated fatty acids. There is absence of trans-fats in natural fats; however, these are formed during partial hydrogenation of oils in industries. The proportion of trans-fats should be cut to a minimum in the daily diet and be kept as low as less than 1% of the total daily calories (for 2,800 calories per day, trans-fats should account for less than 28 calories).

Excessive fat consumption has deleterious effects on the body. Excess fats delay gastric emptying and cause nausea and vomiting. The excess fats irritate the intestinal mucosa and increase motility causing diarrhea. Excess fat intake reduces the digestion of proteins in the intestine.

## WATER

Water is essential for living organisms (Popkin et al. 2010) and it is an essential nutrient (Bourne and Seager 2001).

Water is the inorganic molecule that represents an essential nutrient that is vital for normal maintenance of health and indispensable for the survival of organisms (Jéquier and Constant 2010). Water serves as a universal solvent and an aqueous medium essential for biochemical reactions and metabolic reactions (Iowa State University 2019). It is functionally dynamic for the integrity of plasma membrane and cell structure. Water is indispensable for sustaining the homeostasis of the body and necessary for thermoregulation (Ramsay 1998; Vokes 1987). Water helps in transporting nutrients to body tissues and removing waste materials from body tissues (Panel on Dietary Reference 2005). Water maintains the integrity of extracellular and intracellular fluid compartments. Water serves as a medium in which gas as oxygen is dissolved and transported from the pulmonary alveoli to body tissues while the carbon dioxide is transported from body tissues to the pulmonary alveoli in the dissolved form in water (Royal Society of Chemistry 2019).

Water is the chief structural component of the human body, performing a wide variety of physiological functions. It is necessary for the regulation of body temperature, serves as a fluid component of the extracellular and intracellular compartments, acts as a shock absorber and a solvent. Water functions as the transporter of various organic and inorganic compounds (nutrients and waste products) in the body (Jéquier and Constant 2010; Grandjean et al. 2003); the fluid loss occurs through sweating, urine, stools, and insensible losses from the body.

Water as a nutrient constitutes 60–70% of the total weight of body in the case of a healthy adult person, making up around 49 kg of body weight for the hypothetical adult person whose weight is 70 kg under normal healthy conditions.

The total body water is maintained primarily through a renal mechanism and the phenomenon of constancy of body fluid is called water homeostasis and the human body in the state of normal body fluid is called euhydration. Water as a nutrient is subjected to a state of disturbance when the total body water is depleted owing to loss of body fluid by various causes and the body is said to be in a state of dehydration (hypo-hydration), while an excessive intake of fluid can lead to a state of water intoxication (hyper-hydration).

Input of water is the consumption of fluids either in the form of pure drinking water or as a constituent of the drinks (beverages) and as a component of animal- and plant-based foods (preformed water). Water input also comprises the water derived from the metabolism of macromolecules inside the human body. According to Mellanby (1942), complete oxidation of 100 g of fats yields nearly 110 g of metabolic water, while complete combustion of 100 g of carbohydrates provides 55 g of water.

Lloyd et al. (1978) reported that metabolic water is derived from the oxidation of metabolism of hydrogen-containing compounds or energy-rich nutrients inside the body of living organisms. The oxidation of carbohydrates, proteins, and fats yields nearly 15 g, 10.5 g, and 11.1 g of metabolic water per 100 kcal of energy, respectively.

*Input* refers to fluids consumed as beverages, as either pure water or water contained in drinks, and as part of food (both of which are sometimes collectively called "preformed water"), along with small volumes resulting from the oxidation of food and the breakdown of body tissue ("metabolic water"). The oxidation of 100 g of fat, carbohydrates or proteins will result in 107 g, 55 g, or 41 g of water, respectively (Panel on Dietary Reference Intakes for Electrolytes and Water 2005). Dietary intake of fluids depends on their availability, physiological control (via the thirst center), as well as personal and social factors, such as palatability of drinks and time available for fluid intake.

The World Health Organization (WHO 2005) recommends a total water intake in males as 2.9 L per day and in females as 2.2 L per day. The dietary reference intake of water by the Food and Nutrition Board for males is 3.7 L and 2.7 L for females. Further, it is recommended that around 2.2 L and 3 L of water intake for females and males, respectively, should definitely be derived from beverages (FNB 2005). The European Food Safety Authority recommends the intake of water per day for males as 2.5 L and 2 L for females (EFSA 2010).

Thus, authorities across the world have provided recommendations for total water intake per day. These recommendations are based on the dietary habits, seasonal variation, lifestyle, and condition of the body. Further, it is posited that 20–30% of the total daily water intake should be derived from food, while 70–80% should be obtained from beverages (Jéquier and Constant 2010).

In newborn infants up to the age of six months, the dietary reference intake recommended by the Food and Nutrition Board for the total daily intake of water is 700 ml, which is to be met with exclusive breastfeeding (WHO 2009). The daily water intake for infants aged 7–12 months is 800 mL, for infants aged 1–3 years it is 1.3 L, and for infants aged 4–7 years it is 1.7 L (FNB 2005).

It has been posited that the daily water requirement of children is higher in comparison to adults owing to the higher body surface area of children in relation to their body weight together with restricted renal ability to handle solute loads (Whitmore 2000).

Older people often suffer from dehydration, which has serious repercussions on their health. Dehydration is the result of changes in the structure and function of the kidneys, which affect the ability of the kidneys to sustain normal total body water. There is decrease in the size of the kidneys, a reduction in the flow of blood, and a reduction in the glomerular filtration rate that is chiefly involved in dehydration in the geriatric period (Bennet 2000; Lavizzo-Mourey 1987; Scales 2011).

## MINERALS

Minerals represent the dietary inorganic elements that are necessary for living organisms for multiple functions. This can be calcification of bones and teeth, the structural component of body fluids, serving as a cofactor in enzymatic activity, essentiality in blood coagulation, and in nerve impulse conduction.

The elements carbon, hydrogen, nitrogen, and oxygen are excluded from the category of minerals as these are the structural elements of macronutrients in the human body. Minerals are supplied in a daily diet in which these exist as complex substances. Minerals have to be supplemented in food in which they are deficient in endemic areas, as in the case of iodine, which is supplemented in table salt.

Some minerals are required in large quantities whose Recommended Daily Allowance is higher than 150 mg per day. These minerals are termed *essential minerals*, while the minerals that are required in trace quantity are termed *trace minerals*. The Recommended Daily Allowance of trace minerals is less than 150 mg per day.

The absorption of minerals from the alimentary canal is rapid when these are present in natural form in the food in comparison to the minerals that are supplemented in a diet.

## ESSENTIAL MINERALS

## CALCIUM

Calcium is the most predominant element in the human body.

The human skeleton contains nearly 99% of the total calcium of the body. In an adult person of 70 kg weight, the body contains nearly 1 kg calcium by weight that is contained in the hard tissues of the body in the form of hydroxyapatite crystals. The human skeleton serves as a reservoir of calcium from which calcium can be removed to increase the plasma calcium level or it can be deposited in the body that helps in the remodeling of bones. The calcium is in dynamic equilibrium in the body depending on the calcium needs of the body.

Calcium and calcitriol are essential for the normal mineralization of bones and teeth. Calcium serves as an intracellular signaling molecule to control the cellular functions. Calcium is helpful in the coagulation of blood and is necessary for the transmission of nerve impulse. Calcium is essential for the formation of actin-myosin complex in the skeletal muscles, which is needed in muscle contraction.

The sources of calcium are milk, cheese, yogurt, tofu, and green leafy vegetables like broccoli, fruits, sardines, salmon, and supplemented beverages.

Absorption of calcium is based upon factors that serve as promoters and inhibitors of absorption. Calcitriol, proteins in diet, lactose, and carbohydrates (oligosaccharides) promote the absorption of calcium from the intestinal mucosa. Factors like phytates (in pulses, cereals), oxalates (in beetroot, spinach), phosphoric acid, antacids, and dietary fibers inhibit the absorption of calcium.

## Magnesium

Magnesium is essential as a cofactor in many biochemical reactions and for the synthesis of adenosine triphosphate (ATP) in body.

## Phosphorus

Phosphorus is an essential component of the hard tissues of the body. It is necessary for energy production in the body. It is found in fish, meat, eggs, milk, rice, cereals, and oats.

## Potassium

Potassium is the common electrolyte of intracellular fluid. Its concentration is 140 mEq/L in intracellular fluid (ICF). It is found in tomatoes, sweet potatoes, beans, cereals, lentils, milk, carrots, and oranges.

## Sodium

Sodium is an important mineral of extracellular fluid (ECF). Its concentration is 142 mEq/L in extracellular fluid.

## Sulfur

Sulfur is necessary for the synthesis of amino acids, such as methionine and cysteine. It is found in eggs, meat, onion, garlic, and cabbage.

## TRACE MINERALS

Trace minerals are required in less than 150 mg per day. These serve as cofactors in enzymatic reactions.

### Iron

Iron is a structural component of heme, hemoglobin, myoglobin, and cytochromes. It is found in meat, eggs, jaggery, seafood, and nuts.

### Cobalt

Cobalt is the structural component of vitamin B12.

### Copper

Copper is a necessary component of many enzymes including ceruloplasmin and cytochrome c oxidase. It is found in nuts, grains, legumes, seafood, and oysters.

### Chromium

Chromium is necessary for lipid and glucose metabolism. It is found in grape juice, broccoli, meat, and cereals.

### Iodine

Iodine is essential for the synthesis of thyroid hormones. It prevents goiter. It is found in iodized salt, eggs, and grains.

### Selenium

Selenium is a component of antioxidant glutathione peroxidase. It is found in seafood, nuts, meat, eggs, dairy products, and cereals.

### Zinc

Zinc is essential as a cofactor in the activity of enzymes namely carbonic anhydrase, alcohol dehydrogenase, and carboxypeptidase.

## VITAMINS

### Vitamin A

Vitamin A is a fat-soluble vitamin. It exists in three forms as retinal, retinoic acid, and retinol. It is found in fish, liver, milk and milk products, green leafy vegetables, oranges, carrots, pumpkin, spinach, and mangoes. Its deficiency is responsible for night blindness, keratomalacia, and hyperkeratosis.

### Vitamin D

Vitamin D is a fat-soluble vitamin. It exists in cholecalciferol and ergocalciferol forms. It is found in liver, eggs, meat, and sardines. Its deficiency results in rickets in children and osteomalacia in adults.

### Vitamin E

Vitamin E is a fat-soluble vitamin. It is an antioxidant. It exists in tocopherols and tocotrienols forms. It is found in seed oils, nuts, and fruits. Its deficiency is uncommon.

### Vitamin K

Vitamin K is a fat-soluble vitamin. It is found in green vegetables, egg yolks, and spinach. Its deficiency results in bleeding disorders.

### Vitamin C

Vitamin C is a water-soluble vitamin. It is an antioxidant. It is found in grapes, amla, oranges, and other citrus fruits. Its deficiency results in scurvy.

### Vitamin B1

Vitamin B1 is also called thiamine. It is found in meat, eggs, milk, brown rice, vegetables, and liver. Its deficiency results into beriberi and Wernicke-Korsakoff syndrome.

### Vitamin B2

Vitamin B2 is also called riboflavin. It is found in meat, eggs, milk, brown rice, vegetables, and liver. Its deficiency causes stomatitis, glossitis, and angular cheilitis.

## Vitamin B3

Vitamin B3 is also called niacin. It is found in meat, eggs, milk, brown rice, vegetables, and liver. Its deficiency causes pellagra.

## Vitamin B5

Vitamin B5 is also called pantothenic acid. It is found in broccoli, meat, eggs, and avocadoes. Its deficiency causes paraesthesia in limbs.

## Vitamin B6

Vitamin B6 is also called pyridoxine. It is found in meat, eggs, vegetables, and cereals. Its deficiency causes anemia and peripheral neuropathy.

## Biotin

Biotin is found in raw egg yolks, nuts, vegetables, and fruits. Its deficiency causes dermatitis.

## Folic acid

Folic acid is found in leafy vegetables, cereals, meat, eggs, and fruits. Its deficiency results in megaloblastic anemia.

## Cyanocobalamin

Cyanocobalamin is also called vitamin B12. It is found in meat, eggs, and milk products. Its deficiency results in pernicious anemia.

## PROBIOTICS, PREBIOTICS, AND SYNBIOTICS

An aspect of nutrition that is gaining importance focuses on the prevention of diseases. The word "probiotic" is derived from the Greek that means "in favor of life." Ferdinand Vergin coined the term "probiotic" in 1954 in his article entitled "Anti- und Probiotika," which focused on the comparison of the side effects of the use of antibiotics on the growth of colonic bacteria and the useful effects of selected bacteria on the growth and proliferation of colonic bacteria (Vergin 1954).

Later in 1965, Lilly and Stillwell referred to probiotics as microbes that enhance the growth and proliferation of other microorganisms. Another concept provided by Fuller (1989) mentioned that probiotics are the living microbes that must show beneficial effects on the body of their host. The latest definition was furnished by the Food and Agriculture Organization (FAO) of the United Nations and the World Health Organization (WHO) working group experts in 2002. They described probiotics as live strains of selected microbes that upon oral administration in sufficient amounts provide beneficial effects on the body of their host (FAO 2002).

Probiotics should be safe for the host and have no adverse effects on the host body. The selected strains should not be associated with infectious diseases. The microbes should be resistant to low pH in gastric juices and should be able to withstand host enzymes. The probiotics should be competitive to the colonic microbes and should have antagonistic action against the pathogens in the alimentary canal of the host. The selected strains should be able to colonize and survive in the gut of the host. The probiotics should have genetic stability and should be resistant to the action of bacteriophages.

The probiotic microbes in humans belong to *Lactobacillus*, *Bifidobacterium*, *Enterococcus*, *Streptococcus*, and *Lactococcus* species. Additionally, the microbes of genus *Saccharomyces* are included in the probiotics (Simon 2005).

Probiotics stimulate the growth and proliferation of the colonic commensals for the health benefits of the host. These strains help to maintain a balance between the pathogens and commensals inhabiting the gut of the host. Moreover, the probiotics counteract the pathogenicity of the microbes in the gut that enter with the intake of contaminated food and drinking water. Probiotics inhibit the growth and mitosis of *Clostridium perfringens* (Schoster et al. 2013), *Salmonella* (Carter et al. 2017), *Shigella* (Hussain et al. 2017), *E. coli* (Chingwaru and Vidmar 2017), and *Staphylococcus* (Sikorska and Smoragiewicz 2013) that are implicated in food poisoning.

Studies have proved four modes of action of probiotics in humans. The first method is the antagonistic action, where the probiotics produce the antimicrobial compounds in the gut that counteract the pathogenic organisms and their metabolites (Vandenbergh 1993). The second method is the competitive adherence to the wall of gut of the host (Guillot 2003). Third is the modulation of the immunity of the host (Isolauri et al. 2001). The fourth method is the inhibition of growth and mitosis of pathogens and their toxins in the gut of the host (Brandao et al. 1998).

In 1995, Gibson and Roberfroid defined "prebiotics" as the non-digested foodstuff that, after activation by the colonic microbes, helps in the improvement in the health status of the host. In 2004, the definition of prebiotics was refined as strictly selected and fermented foodstuff that could alter the composition and microbial activity of colonic commensals for the health benefits of the host (Gibson et al. 2004).

Later in 2007, the FAO and WHO experts mentioned that prebiotics are the non-living foodstuffs that provide health benefits to the host linked with the alteration in the composition and activity of the colonic microbes (FAO 2007).

Prebiotics enhance the growth of gut microbes. Cereals, fruits, vegetables, and salad are good sources of prebiotics. Other sources could be tomatoes, berries, bananas, asparagus, onions, garlic, green vegetables, legumes, and oats (Crittenden and Playne 2008). The synthetic prebiotics could be lactulose, cyclodextrins, fructooligosaccharides, maltooligosaccharides, and inulin.

Prebiotics have inherent resistance to the low pH in stomach, bile salts, and proteases in the gut of the host. They also promote the growth of the friendly microbes in the gut that provide health benefits to the host. Conversely, prebiotics retain a large amount of water in the gut that may enhance peristaltic movements of the gut. Prebiotics also decrease the pH of the gut. These effects may cause diarrhea and flatulence upon the intake of large amount of prebiotics.

The mechanism of action of prebiotics is the increased synthesis of short-chain fatty acids in the body. These compounds control the activity of lipogenic enzymes of the liver. The butyric acid that is produced in response to the prebiotics could modulate the acetylation of histones.

The prebiotics could increase the white blood cell (WBC) count in the gut and associated lymphoid tissues and blood circulation. The further synthesis of immunoglobulin A (IgA) is increased through the activity of gut-associated lymphoid tissues in the body. IgA enhances the activity of macrophages.

In 1995, Gibson and Roberfroid coined the term "synbiotic" to explain the synergistic functioning of probiotics and prebiotics in the body of the host. Synbiotics possess the properties of probiotics and prebiotics so that the possibility of survival of probiotics should be increased in the alimentary canal of the host.

## REFERENCES

Ahrens, R. (1977) William Prout (1785–1850): A biographical sketch. *Journal of Nutrition* 107(1): 15–23.

American Association of Cereal Chemists (1998) The definition of dietary fibers. Available at: www.aaccnet.org/initiatives/definitions/Documents/DietaryFiber/DFDef.pdf

American Association of Cereal Chemists (2001) The definition of dietary fiber: An AACC Report. *Cereals Food World* 46(3): 112–126.

American Diabetes Association (2013) Standards of medical care in diabetes, 2013. *Diabetes Care* 12(S1): S11–S66.

Bay, A. (2012) *Beriberi in Modern Japan: The Making of a National Disease.* New York: University of Rochester Press.

Bennett, J.A. (2000) Dehydration: Hazards and benefits. *Geriatric Nursing* 21(2): 84–88.

Bourne, L.T. and Seager, J.R. (2001) Water: The neglected nutrient. *South African Journal of Clinical Nutrition* 14(3): S64–S77.

Brandao, R.L., Castro, I.M., Bambirra, E.A., Amaral, S.C., Fietto, L.G., and Tropia, M.J.M. (1998) Intracellular signal triggered by cholera toxin in *Saccharomyces boulardii* and *Saccharomyces cerevisiae*. *Applied Environmental Microbiology* 64: 564–568.

British Nutrition Foundation (2018) Dietary fibres. Available at: www.nutrition.org.uk/nutritionscience/nutrients-food-and-ingredients/dietary-fibre.html?limitstart=0

Calder, P.C. (2016) Docosahexaenoic acid. *Annals of Nutrition and Metabolism* S1: 7–21.

Cambridge Dictionary (2019) Nutrition. Available at: https://dictionary. cambridge.org/dictionary/english/nutrition

Carter, A., Adams, M., La Ragione, R.M., and Woodward, M.J. (2017) Colonisation of poultry by *Salmonella enteritidis* S1400 is reduced by combined administration of *Lactobacillus salivarius* 59 and *Enterococcus faecium* PXN-33. *Veterinary Microbiology* 199: 100–107.

Calder, P.C. (2016) Docosahexaenoic acid. *Annals of Nutrition and Metabolism* S1: 7–21.

Center for Food Safety, Government of Hong Kong (2019) Nutrients introduction. Available at: www.cfs.gov.hk/english/nutrient/ nutrient.php

Chingwaru, W. and Vidmar, J. (2017) Potential of Zimbabwean commercial probiotic products and strains of *Lactobacillus plantarum* as prophylaxis and therapy against diarrhoea caused by *Escherichia coli* in children. *Asian Pacific Journal of Tropical Medicine* 10: 57–63.

Crittenden, R. and Playne, M.J. (2008) Nutrition news: Facts and functions of prebiotics, probiotics and synbiotics. In Y.K. Lee and S. Salminen (eds.), *Handbook of Probiotics and Prebiotics*. Hoboken, NJ, and Manhattan, KS: Wiley-Interscience and Kansas State University, pp. 535–582.

Eijkman, C. (1929) Nobel Lecture: The Nobel Prize in Physiology or Medicine. Available at: www.nobelprize.org/nobel_prizes/medicine/laureates/1929/eijkman-lecture.html

Elena, C. (2006) Fortified foods took out rickets. *Los Angeles Times*.

Elliott, J. (2007) Elsie—Mother of the modern loaf. *BBC News*.

Evans, H.M., Emerson, O.H., and Emerson G.A. (1936) The isolation from wheat germ oil of an alcohol, a-tocopherol, having the properties of vitamin E. *Journal of Biological Chemistry* 113(1): 319–332.

European Food Safety Authority (2010) Scientific opinion on dietary reference values for water. *EFSA Journal* 8(3):1459. Available at: www. efsa.europa.eu/it/ scdocs/doc/1459.pdf

Food and Agriculture Organization (FAO) (2002) *Guidelines for the Evaluation of Probiotics in Food*. London: FAO/WHO.

Food and Agriculture Organization (FAO) (2007) *Technical Meeting on Prebiotics: Food Quality and Standards Service (AGNS)*. Rome: FAO.

Food and Agriculture Organization (FAO) (2019) Dietary carbohydrate and disease. Available at: www.fao.org/3/W8079E/w8079e09.htm

Food and Nutrition Board (2005) Dietary reference intakes for water, potassium, sodium, chloride, and sulphate. Available at: http://print.nap.edu/pdf/0309091691/pdf_image/143.pdf

Fuller, R. (1989) Probiotics in man and animals. *Journal of Applied Microbiology* 66: 365–378.

Gaesser, G.A. (2007) Carbohydrate quantity and quality in relation to body mass index. *Journal of the American Dietetic Association* 107(10): 1768–1780.

Gibson, R.G. and Roberfroid, M.B. (1995) Dietary modulation of the human colonic microbiota: Introducing the concept of prebiotics. *Journal of Nutrition* 125: 1401–1412.

Gibson, G.R., Probert, H.M., van Loo, J., Rastall, R.A., and Roberfroid, M. (2004) Dietary modulation of the human colonic microbiota: Updating the concept of the prebiotics. *Nutrition Research Reviews* 17: 259–275.

Guillot, J.F. (2003) Probiotic feed additives. *Journal of Veterinary Pharmacology and Therapeutics* 26: 52–55.

Gunness, P. and Gidley, M.J. (2010) Mechanisms underlying the cholesterol-lowering properties of soluble dietary fibre polysaccharides. *Food & Function* 1(2): 149–155.

Grandjean, A.C., Reimers, K.J., and Buyckx, M.E. (2003) Hydration: Issues for the 21st century. *Nutrition Reviews* 61(8): 261–271.

Gratzer, W. (2005) *Terrors of the Table: The Curious History of Nutrition.* Oxford: Oxford University Press.

Hipsley, E.H. (1953) Dietary "fibre" and pregnancy toxaemia. *British Medical Journal* 2: 420–422.

Hopkins, F.G. (1912) Feeding experiments illustrating the importance of accessory factors in normal dietaries. *Journal of Physiology* 44(5–6): 425–460.

Hussain, S.A., Patil, G.R., Reddi, S., Yadav, V., Pothuraju, R., Singh, R.R.B., and Kapila, S. (2017) Aloe vera (*Aloe barbadensis* Miller) supplemented probiotic lassi prevents *Shigella* infiltration from epithelial barrier into systemic blood flow in mice model. *Microbial Pathogenesis* 102: 143–147.

Institute of Medicine (2001) *Panel on the Definition of Dietary Fiber and the Standing Committee on the Scientific Evaluation of Dietary Reference Intakes.* Washington, DC: National Academies Press.

Iowa State University (2019) Water as solvent. Available at: http://agron-www.agron.iastate.edu/courses/Agron541/classes/review/water/1.4.html

Isolauri, E., Sutas, Y., Kankaanpaa, P., Arvilommi, H., and Salminen, S. (2001) Probiotics: Effects on immunity. *American Journal of Clinical Nutrition* 73: 444–450.

Jéquier, E. and Constant, F. (2010) Water as an essential nutrient: The physiological basis of hydration. *European Journal of Clinical Nutrition* 64: 115–123.

Kafatos, A. and Hatzis, C. (2008) *Clinical Nutrition for Medical Students.* Rethymnon: University of Crete.

Kenneth, J.C. (2003) A short history of nutritional science: Part 1 (1785–1885). *Journal of Nutrition* 133(3): 638–645.

Kunzmann, A.T., Coleman, H.G., Huang, W.-Y., Kitahara, C.M., Cantwell, M.M., and Berndt, S.I. (2005) Dietary fiber intake and risk of colorectal cancer and incident and recurrent adenoma in the Prostate, Lung, Colorectal, and Ovarian Cancer Screening Trial. *American Journal of Clinical Nutrition* 102(4): 881–890.

Lavizzo-Mourey, R.J. (1987) Dehydration in the elderly: A short review. *Journal of the National Medical Association* 79(10): 1033–1038.

Lilly, D.M. and Stillwell, R.H. (1965) Probiotics: Growth promoting factors produced by microorganisms. *Science* 147: 747–748.

Lipkin, M., Reddy, B., Newmark, H., and Lamprecht, S.A. (1999) Dietary factors in human colorectal cancer. *Annual Review of Nutrition* 19: 545–586.

Lloyd, L.E., McDonald, B.E., and Crampton, E.W. (1978) Water and its metabolism. In *Fundamentals of Nutrition*, 2nd ed. San Francisco: W.H. Freeman, pp. 22–35.

Low, M. (2005) *Building a Modern Japan: Science, Technology, and Medicine in the Meiji Era and Beyond.* London: Palgrave Macmillan.

Magendie, F. (1816) Sur les propriétés nutritives des substances qui ne ntiennent pas d' azote. *Annali di chimica* 3: 66–77, 408–410.

McClean, F.C. and Budy, A.M. (1964) Vitamin A, vitamin D, cartilage, bones, and teeth. *Vitamins and Hormones,* 21: 51–68.

Mellanby, K. (1942) Metabolic water and desiccation. *Nature* 150: 21.

Nathani, N. (2013) An appraisal of the concept of diet and dietetics in Ayurveda. *Asian Journal of Modern and Ayurvedic Medical Science* 2: 1–9. Available at: www.ajmams.com/viewpaper.aspx?pcode= ef5cc006-6583-4806-b293-7d170f36d956

National Institutes of Health (2019) Omega-3-Fatty acid. Available at: https://ods.od.nih.gov/factsheets/Omega3FattyAcids-HealthProfessional/

Osborne, T.B. and Mendel, L.B. (1914) Amino acids in nutrition and growth. *Journal of Biological Chemistry,* 17: 325–349.

Panel on Dietary Reference Intakes for Electrolytes and Water (2005) *Dietary Reference Intakes for Water, Potassium, Sodium, Chloride, and Sulfate.* Washington, DC: National Academies Press.

Payne-Palacio, J.R. and Canter, D.D. (2014) *The Profession of Dietetics.* Burlington, MA: Jones & Bartlett Learning.

Peters, J.C. (1991) Tryptophan nutrition and metabolism: An overview. In R. Schwarcz, S.N. Young, and R.R. Brown (eds.), *Kynurenine and Serotonin Pathways: Advances in Experimental Medicine and Biology.* Boston, MA: Springer.

Popkin, B.M., D'Anci, K.E., and Rosenberg, I.H. (2010) Water, hydration and health. *Nutrition Reviews* 68(8): 439–458.

Post, R.E., Mainous, A.G. III, King, D.E., and Simpson, K.N. (2012) Dietary fiber for the treatment of type 2 diabetes mellitus: A meta-analysis. *Journal of the American Board of Family Medicine* 12: 16–23.

Ramsay, D.J. (1998) Homeostatic control of water balance. In M.J. Arnaud (ed.), *Hydration throughout Life.* Montrouge: John Libbey Eurotext, pp. 9–18.

Ricciotti, E. and FitzGerald, G.A. (2011) Prostaglandins and inflammation. *Arteriosclerosis, Thrombosis, and Vascular Biology* 31(5): 986–1000.

Rose, W.C. (1957) The amino acid requirements of adult man. *Nutrition Abstracts and Reviews* 27: 631–647.

Royal Society of Chemistry (2019) Gas exchange. Available at: www.rsc.org/Education/Teachers/Resources/cfb/gas.htm

Samra, R.A. (2010) Fats and satiety. In J.P. Montmayeur and J. le Coutre (eds.), *Fat Detection: Taste, Texture, and Post Ingestive Effects.* Boca Raton, FL: CRC Press/Taylor & Francis.

Scales, K. (2011) Use of hypodermoclysis to manage dehydration. *Nursing Older People* 23(5): 16–22.

Schoster, A., Kokotovic, B., Permin, A., Pedersen, P.D., Dal Bello, F., and Guardabassi, L. (2013) In vitro inhibition of *Clostridium difficile* and *Clostridium perfringens* by commercial probiotic strains. *Anaerobe* 20: 36–41.

Seguin, A. and Lavoisier, A.L. (1789) Premier mémoire sur la transpiration des animaux. *Mémoires de l'Académie royale des sciences* 179: 601–661.

Sengupta, S., Muir, J.G., and Gibson, P.R. (2006) Does butyrate protect from colorectal cancer? *Journal of Gastroenterology & Hepatology* 21: 209–218.

Shastri, A. (ed.) (2003) *Sushruta: Sushruta Samhita with Ayurveda Tattva Sandipika Hindi Commentary*, 14th ed. Varanasi: Chaukhambha Sanskrit Sansthan.

Sikorska, H. and Smoragiewicz, W. (2013) Role of probiotics in the prevention and treatment of methicillin-resistant *Staphylococcus aureus* infections. *International Journal of Antimicrobial Agents* 42: 475–481.

Simon, O. (2005) Micro-organisms as feed additives—probiotics. *Advances in Pork Production* 16: 161–167.

Smith, R. (2004) Let food be thy medicine... *BMJ* 328(7433).

Trowell, H. (1972) Ischemic heart disease and dietary fibre. *American Journal of Clinical Nutrition* 25: 926–932.

U.S. Department of Agriculture (2019) USDA MyPlate & Food Pyramid Resources. Available at: www.nal.usda.gov/fnic

U.S. Department of Health and Human Services and Department of Agriculture (2005a) Dietary Guidelines for Americans 2005 (PDF). Available at: https://health.gov/sites/default/files/2020-01/DGA2005.pdf

U.S. Department of Health and Human Services and Department of Agriculture (2005b) How Much Physical Activity Is Needed? Available at: www.choosemyplate.gov/resources/physical-activity-amount

U.S. National Library of Medicine, National Institutes of Health (1998) Joint Collection Development Policy. Available at: http://www.nlm.nih.gov/pubs/cd_hum.nut.html#2.

U.S. National Library of Medicine, National Institutes of Health (2019) Joint Collection Development Policy: Human Nutrition and Food. Available at: www.nlm.nih.gov/pubs/cd_hum.nut.htm

Vandenbergh, P.A. (1993) Lactic acid bacteria, their metabolic products and interference with microbial growth. *FEMS Microbiology Reviews* 12: 221–238.

Vergin, F. (1954) Anti- und Probiotika. *Hipokrates* 25: 116–119.

Vokes, T. (1987) Water homeostasis. *Annual Review of Nutrition* 7: 383–406.

Whitmore, S.J. (2000) Water, electrolytes and acid-base balance. In L.K. Mahan and S. Escott-Stump (eds.), *Krause's Food, Nutrition and Diet Therapy*. Philadelphia: WB Saunders Company, pp. 151–163.

Whitney, E. and Rolfes, S.R. (2013) *Understanding Nutrition*, 13th ed. Wadsworth: Cengage Learning.

Willcock, E.G. and Hopkins, F.G. (1906) The importance of individual amino acids in metabolism: Observations on the effect of adding tryptophan to a diet in which zein is the sole nitrogenous constituent. *Journal of Psychology* 35: 88–102.

Willett, W.C. with Skerrett, P.J. (2005) *Eat, Drink, and Be Healthy: The Harvard Medical School Guide to Healthy Eating.* New York: Free Press, Simon & Schuster.

Windaus, A. (1928) Constitution of Sterols and Their Connection with Other Substances Occurring in Nature. Available at: www. nobelprize.org/uploads/2018/06/windaus-lecture.pdf

World Health Organization (2005) Nutrients in drinking water. Available at: www. who.int/water_sanitation_health/dwq/nutrientsindw.pdf

World Health Organization (2009) Infant and young child feeding. Available at: www.who.int/nutrition/publications/infantfeeding/ 9789241597494/en/ index.html

World Health Organization (2019) Nutrition. Available at: www.who.int/ topics/nutrition/en/

Wolf, G. (2004) The discovery of vitamin D: The contribution of Adolf Windaus. *Journal of Nutrition* 134(6): 1299–1302.

Young, F.G. (1957) Claude Bernard and the discovery of glycogen. *British Medical Journal* 1(5033): 1431–1437.

# CHAPTER 2

# Biochemical Parameters and Protein-Energy Malnutrition

## EPIDEMIOLOGY

According to the World Health Organization, protein-energy malnutrition (PEM) is defined as the disparity between the intake of energy and/or proteins and the requirement of body tissues to maintain normal growth and development.

PEM is the major health hazard affecting the nutritional status of children below the age of five years. There are three types: *kwashiorkor*, which is mainly the protein malnutrition, while *marasmus* is basically the deficiency of calories intake, and *marasmic kwashiorkor* is characterized by the deficiency of intake of protein as well as calories and represents the severe type of malnutrition.

Depending upon the WHO Global Database on Child Growth involving the child population below the age of five years in developing countries, de Onis et al. (1993) reported the worldwide prevalence of PEM in 79 countries in the period between 1980 and 1992 in Africa, Latin America, Asia, and Oceania. It was reported that more than a third of the child population of the world is affected with PEM, involving wasting, stunting, and being underweight. The authors further reported that the prevalence of PEM in Latin America was either low or moderate, while in Asian countries, the prevalence of PEM was very high, and further iterated that the African countries witnessed the low to high prevalence of PEM.

According to a report by the WHO (2011), each year around 9 million children under the age of five years die owing to malnutrition in developing countries. A further report indicated that 20–30% of severely malnourished children under five die in hospitals in developed countries during treatment (Monte 2000).

## CLINICAL MANIFESTATIONS OF PROTEIN-ENERGY MALNUTRITION

### Kwashiorkor

Kwashiorkor is a severe form of protein malnutrition that is predominantly characterized by presence of edema and hepatomegaly in the affected children.

Kwashiorkor is characterized by intake of adequate amount of calories without supplementation of sufficient quantity of protein in the diet (Gupta 2019). It is a protein deficiency nutritional disorder that arises from the intake of a carbohydrate-rich diet with low protein components.

It was Jamaican pediatrician Cicely Williams who first mentioned the name kwashiorkor in the scientific community in her article that was published in *Lancet* in 1935 (Williams 1983). According to the Merriam Webster Dictionary (2019), the word is derived from the Ga language from coastal Ghana. It signifies the health condition of the older child who was weaned from mother's milk after the birth of the younger sibling. It is the sickness of the older baby.

Kwashiorkor is manifested by the color change and thinning of the hair, loss of pigmentation in the skin, fatigue, loss of muscle mass, frequent episodes of diarrhea, poor growth of body, weight loss, edema over the ankles, feet, and abdomen, compromised immunity, frequent infections, and hepatomegaly (Gupta 2019). The condition exerts prolonged deleterious effects on the growth and development of the affected children.

Kwashiorkor is the sequela of a protein-deficit diet for a prolonged period. The protein deficiency in the body is responsible for diminished oncotic pressure in the vascular compartment. This leads to collection of fluid in the interstitial tissues and formation of pitting edema over the ankles and feet. The distention of abdomen due to retention of fluid is called ascites.

## Marasmus

Marasmus is another severe form of nutritional disorder characterized by a deficiency in calorie intake. The prevalence of marasmus is higher below one year of age in infants while the prevalence of kwashiorkor is higher after the age of one (Olaf and Krawinkel 2005). Marasmus can be differentiated from kwashiorkor in deficiency of calories including proteins, while in the latter condition the child suffers from the exclusive deficiency of proteins.

In kwashiorkor, edema and hepatomegaly along with the ascites are common features that are distinguished from the marasmus, in which muscular atrophy and fat mobilization in the subcutaneous layer are the main characteristics (Olaf and Krawinkel 2005; Appleton and Vanbergen 2013).

The concrete differentiation between the two disorders has little practical value as the clinical manifestations of both disorders merge with each other. It had been reported by Jelliffe (1959) in Asia, South Africa, Central and South America, and the Caribbean that children presented with mixed clinical manifestations of the two disorders. This resulted in the emergence of the protein-energy malnutrition term, marasmic kwashiorkor.

The word *marasmus* is derived from the Greek word, "marasmus" that signifies wasting.

## CLINICAL MANIFESTATIONS

Marasmus is specifically characterized by wasting, muscular atrophy, weight loss, and loss of fat in the subcutaneous layer. The child with marasmus is often younger than a kwashiorkor child. The marasmic child has a deficiency in weight and height. Moreover, the occurrence of edema and hepatomegaly are absent in the marasmic child. The color of skin is often normal with brittle hair. The marasmic child is often hungry and crying.

The marasmic child suffers from anemia, dehydration, and pyrexia.

## ROLE OF SERUM PROTEIN BIOMARKERS IN DIAGNOSIS OF PROTEIN-ENERGY MALNUTRITION

### Serum Albumin

Serum albumin is an important plasma protein that remains circulating in the bloodstream. It is the significant and initial biomarker in protein-energy malnutrition in children and adults.

It has been used in the assessment of malnutrition in the non-hospitalized and hospitalized child populations. Hypoalbuminemia is associated with malnutrition and both conditions predispose to a higher prevalence of mortality in children (Masood and Sanober 1984).

According to Seltzer et al. (1981), hypoalbuminemia is linked to a decrease in the number of lymphocytes and both factors increase the prevalence of morbidity in the hospitalized population of children. The albumin is the plasma protein that is synthesized in the liver. Its plasma concentration is dependent on its synthesis, degradation, and volume of distribution. The albumin is distributed into the extracellular and intracellular compartments in the body. The concentration of the intravascular pool of albumin is maintained. In the stage of liver inflammation or starvation, the synthesis of albumin in liver is decreased and, hence, the albumin fraction of the vascular compartment is declined. As a compensatory mechanism, albumin is mobilized from the extravascular compartment to inside the vascular compartment so as to stabilize the concentration of the serum albumin. Moreover, the biological half-life period of albumin is 20 days. Owing to these factors, the serum albumin value remains fairly static and the concentration of vascular pool of albumin is not affected by the acute malnutrition, and serum albumin is not sensitive biomarker to detect the wasting in children. Furthermore, the prolonged intake of protein deficiency and calorie-rich diet results in the decreased concentration of albumin in the extravascular and vascular compartments that leads to hypoalbuminemia. This condition manifests as kwashiorkor. However, intake of a calorie-deficient but protein-containing diet results in the loss of body weight and depletion in the storage of energy that manifests as a loss of skeletal muscle. This condition is called marasmus.

Serum albumin concentration of 3.5 g/100 mL is considered as normal value in children. A fall in serum albumin value for mild PEM is between 2.8 g/100 mL and 3.5 g/100 mL (Grant et al. 1981; Masood and Sanober 1984), while values between 2.1 g/ 100 mL, and 2.7 g/100 mL and less than 2.1 g/100 mL are indicative of the moderate and severe forms of protein-energy malnutrition, respectively (Grant et al. 1981; Masood and Sanober 1984).

## Serum Prealbumin

Serum prealbumin is also referred to as transthyretin. It is synthesized in the liver and is involved in the transport of thyroid hormones. In assessing malnutrition, the concentration of serum prealbumin below 10 mg/100 mL is significant (Beck and Rosenthal 2002). It is an important biomarker in children and elderly patients. (Takeda et al. 2003). It has a shorter half-life period (two days) compared to albumin (Takeda et al. 2003). It is a more sensitive biomarker for protein depletion than albumin. Prealbumin concentration is highly sensitive to any alteration in the concentration of protein in the body as in protein-energy malnutrition (Takeda et al. 2003).

According to Dellière and Cynober (2017), a concentration of prealbumin below 0.11 g/1 L is linked to a high mortality rate and increased duration of hospitalization of patients. Furthermore, the authors asserted that increased loss of prealbumin concentration below 0.04 g/1 L per week showed inadequate nutritional therapy (Dellière and Cynober 2017).

## Transferrin

Transferrin is a glycoprotein that transports ferric iron in the circulation. It is produced in the liver and has a biological half-life period of ten days, which is comparatively shorter than albumin (Shetty et al. 1979). Transferrin protein is more rapidly activated in the decrease in the concentration of protein in the body than the serum albumin. The concentration of transferrin is reduced in conditions of severe protein-energy malnutrition. Moreover, the diagnostic value of transferrin is not equivocally established in the diagnosis of mild, moderate, and subclinical cases of malnutrition (Bharadwaj et al. 2016).

Few authors labeled transferrin as useful in assessing malnutrition, although others contraindicated its use in nutritional assessment (Roza et al. 1984).

In the condition of deficiency of iron in the body, the concentration of transferrin is increased, whereas in the condition of iron overload, its concentration is decreased. The serum transferrin concentration is decreased in children who are suffering from malnutrition. In children who are critically ill, the concentration of serum transferrin along with the level of serum prealbumin are elevated in nutritional therapy. However, serum transferrin is not a good biomarker to assess mild malnutrition in children.

Serum transferrin increased in parallel to prealbumin during nutritional intervention in critically ill children (Briassoulis et al. 2001). Serum levels decrease in the setting of severe malnutrition, but this marker has been found to be unreliable in the assessment of mild malnutrition and of fat-free mass in a group of elderly Italian patients (Sergi et al. 2006).

## Serum Insulin-Like Growth Factor 1

Insulin-like growth factor (IGF) is also called somatomedin C. It is the peptide hormone that is synthesized in the liver and has a substantive role in the growth of children. It exerts an anabolic effect on the body of adults. Structurally, it is composed of 70 amino acid residues and three intra-chain disulfide bridges (Jansen et al. 1983).

Growth hormone activates the release of somatomedin C from the liver. It is the universal growth factor in children. It has a biological half-life period of 24 hours and remains in blood circulation, bound to one binding protein out of six binding proteins (IGFBP). IGFBP-3 is the most predominant binding protein that binds nearly 80% of the IGF in blood circulation. There is a ratio of 1:1 between IGF and IGFBP-3, which in turn is controlled by insulin (Christoffersen et al. 1994).

Starvation and fasting conditions decline the plasma concentration of IGF, while the intake of food and nutrition therapy raise the level of IGF in plasma.

There is a strict correlation between the intake of energy and plasma IGF levels. According to Isley et al. (1983), somatomedin C is a reliable biomarker for protein-energy malnutrition in elderly patients and children.

Isley et al. (1983) tested the somatomedin C plasma levels in five adult patients who first fasted for five days and then were fed diets of different compositions. It was found that serum IGF levels declined from a mean value of 1.85 ± 0.39 U per mL before the time of fasting to 0.67 ± 0.16 U per mL by the time of breakfast. Further, the authors confirmed a rise in the serum IGF levels in the patients after refeeding for the next five days, which was 1.26 ± 0.20 U per mL (Isley et al. 1983).

According to López-Hellin et al. (2002), the plasma level of IGF-1 is not affected by inflammation in the organs or body. It was concluded that retinol-binding protein and transthyretin are influenced by the stress period after surgery and, hence, are inadequate to monitor nutritional assessment (López-Hellin et al. 2002). Contrarily, IGF-1 is not affected by the stress period of surgery, it is a sensitive biomarker, which assesses the effect of nutritional therapy in post-operative patients. Moreover, the plasma level of IGF-1 is altered by liver disease, renal disease, and burns (Shenkin et al. 1996).

Unterman et al. (1985) conducted a study to assess the efficacy of IGF-1 serum levels in monitoring the nutritional status of malnourished patients. They observed the serum somatomedin C levels in 28 patients before the start of therapy, which were found to be lowered by 38% of the normal value. It was observed that serum somatomedin C level was the lowest in the kwashiorkor-marasmus condition (25% of normal condition), while it was 51% of the normal condition in kwashiorkor and 57% of the normal condition in marasmus. Unterman et al. (1985) correlated serum somatomedin C, serum transferrin, serum albumin, and lymphocyte count and concluded that somatomedin C was related to the intake of calories and proteins in 20 patients. They also inferred that serum IGF-1 could be the sensitive biomarker for protein-energy malnutrition and to assess the effect of nutritional therapy.

At the age of 18 years, the median plasma IGF-I level is 374.1 ng/mL, and it declines with age advancement (Zhu et al. 2017).

## Serum Nesfatin-1

Nesfatin-1 is a peptide hormone that is secreted in the hypothalamus in humans. It plays a key role in the regulation of food intake and calorie homeostasis. A rise in the serum nesfatin-1 level leads to diminished intake of food and decline in hunger and decrease in storage of tissue fat.

Acar et al. (2018) conducted a study to find out the effect of nesfatin-1 on the anthropometric indices and metabolic parameters in 37 underweight (idiopathic chronic malnutrition) and 38 normal weight healthy children. The authors found serum nesfatin-1 levels significantly higher in the 37 underweight children in comparison to the healthy children.

Acar et al. (2018) concluded there is strong correlation of serum nesfatin-1 level with malnutrition and parametric indices in children. The authors inferred that nesfatin-1 levels could be implicated in the initiation and pathogenesis of malnutrition by the inhibition of food intake in children.

## Urinary 3-Methylhistidine

3-Methylhistidine is the histidine molecule that undergoes post-translational modification. Urinary 3-methylhistidine concentration is a sensitive biomarker of protein catabolism in the skeletal muscles in humans. It is almost free from the renal function in comparison to the creatinine.

Nagabhushan and Narasinga Rao (1978) estimated the 24-hour urinary excretion of 3-methylhistidine among children suffering from moderate and severe forms of protein-energy malnutrition. The values were recorded pre- and post-treatment. The authors observed a decline in the excretion of 3-methylhistidine in children who suffered from severe protein-energy malnutrition, and they further commented that 3-methylhistidine excretion was increased post-treatment. Nagabhushan and Narasinga Rao (1978) concluded qualitative and quantitative fluctuations in 3-methylhistidine metabolism are implicated in protein-energy malnutrition.

## REFERENCES

Acar, S., Çatlı, G., Küme, T., Tuhan, H., Gürsoy Çalan, Ö., Demir, K., Böber, E., and Abaci, A (2018) Increased concentrations of serum nesfatin-1 levels in childhood with idiopathic chronic malnutrition. *Turkish Journal of Medical Sciences* 48: 378–385.

Appleton, A. and Vanbergen, O. (2013) *Crash Course: Metabolism and Nutrition*, 4th ed. Maryland Heights, MI: Mosby.

Beck, F.K. and Rosenthal, T.C. (2002) Prealbumin: A marker for nutritional evaluation. *American Family Physician* 65: 1575–1580.

Bharadwaj, S., Ginoya, S., Tandon, P., Gohel, T.D., Guirguis, J., Vallabh, H., Jevenn, A., and Hanouneh, I. (2016) Malnutrition: Laboratory markers vs nutritional assessment. *Gastroenterology Report* 4: 272–280.

Briassoulis, G., Zavras, N., and Hatzis, T. (2001) Malnutrition, nutritional indices, and early enteral feeding in critically ill children. *Nutrition* 17: 548–557.

Christoffersen, C.T., Bornfeldt, K.E., Rotella, C.M., Gonzales, N., Vissing, H., and Shymko, R.M. (1994) Negative cooperativity in the insulin-like growth factor-I receptor and a chimeric IGF-I/insulin receptor. *Endocrinology* 135(1): 472–475.

Dellière, S. and Cynober, L.(2017) Is transthyretin a good marker of nutritional status? *Clinical Nutrition* 36: 364–370.

de Onis, M., Monteiro, C., Akré, J., and Clugston, G. (1993) The worldwide magnitude of protein-energy malnutrition: An overview from the WHO Global Database on Child Growth. *Bulletin of the World Health Organization* 71(6): 703–712.

Gupta, A. (2019) *Comprehensive Biochemistry for Dentistry: Textbook for Dental Students.* Boston, MA: Springer.

Grant, J.P., Custer, P.B., and Thurlow, J. (1981) Current techniques of nutritional assessment. *Surgical Clinics of North America* 61:437–463.

Isley, W.L., Underwood, L.E., and Clemmons, D.R. (1983) Dietary components that regulate serum somatomedin-C concentrations in humans. *Journal of Clinical Investigation* 71(2): 175–182.

Jansen, M., van Schaik, F.M., Ricker, A.T., Bullock, B., Woods, D.E., Gabbay, K.H., Nussbaum, A.L., Sussenbach, J.S., and Van den Brande, J.L. (1983) Sequence of cDNA encoding human insulin-like growth factor I precursor. *Nature* 306(5943): 609–611.

López-Hellin, J., Baena-Fustegueras, J.A., Schwartz-Riera, S., and García-Arumí, E. (2002) Usefulness of short-lived proteins as nutritional indicators surgical patients. *Clinical Nutrition* 21:119–125.

Masood, H. and Sanober, Q.H. (1984) Assessment of protein-calorie malnutrition. *Clinical Chemistry* 30(8): 1286–1299.

Merriam Webster Dictionary (2019) Kwashiorkor. Available at: www.merriam-webster.com/dictionary/kwashiorkor

Monte, C.M.G. (2000) Malnutrition: A secular challenge to child nutrition. *Jornal de Pediatria* 76(S3): 285–297.

Nagabhushan, V.S. and Narasinga Rao, B.S. (1978) Studies on 3-methylhistidine metabolism in children with protein-energy malnutrition. *American Journal of Clinical Nutrition* 31(8): 1322–1327.

Olaf, M. and Krawinkel, M. (2005) Malnutrition and health in developing countries. *Canadian Medical Association Journal* 173(3): 279–286.

Roza, A.M., Tuitt, D., and Shizgal, H.M. (1984) Transferrin—a poor measure of nutritional status. *Journal of Parenteral and Enteral Nutrition* 8: 523–528.

Seltzer, M.H., Fletcher, H.S., Slocum, B.A., and Engler, P.E. (1981) Instant nutritional assessment in the intensive care unit. *Journal of Parenteral and Enteral Nutrition* 5(1): 70–72.

Sergi, G., Coin, A., Enzi, G., Volpato, S., Inelmen, E.M., Buttarello, M., Peloso, M., Mulone, S., Marin, S., and Bonometto, P. (2006) Role of visceral proteins in detecting malnutrition in the elderly. *European Journal of Clinical Nutrition* 60: 203–209.

Shenkin, A., Cederblad, G., Elia, M., and Isaksson, B. (1996) Laboratory assessment of protein-energy status. *Clinica Chimica Acta* 253: S5–S9.

Shetty, P.S., Jung, R., Watrasiewics, K., and James, W.P. (1979) Rapid turnover transport proteins: An index of subclinical protein energy malnutrition. *Lancet* 2: 230–232.

Takeda, H., Ishihama, K., Fukui, T., Fujishima, S., Orii, T., Nakazawa, Y., Shu, H.J., and Kawara, S. (2003) Significance of rapid turnover proteins in protein-losing gastroenteropathy. *Hepatogastroenterology* 50(54): 1963–1965.

Unterman, T.G., Vazquez, R.M., Slas, A.J., Martyn, P.A., and Phillips, L.S. (1985) Nutrition and somatomedin. XIII. Usefulness of somatomedin-C in nutritional assessment. *American Journal of Medicine* 78: 228–234.

Williams, C.D. (1983) Fifty years ago. Archives of Diseases in Childhood 1933. A nutritional disease of childhood associated with a maize diet. *Archives of Disease in Childhood* 58(7): 550–560.

World Health Organization (2011) Child mortality. Available at: www.who.int/pmnch/media/press_materials/fs/fs_mdg4_childmortality/en/

Zhu, H. , Xu, Y., Gong, F., Shan, G., Yang, H., Xu, K., Zhang, D., Cheng, X., Zhang, Z., Chen, S., Wang, L., and Pan, H. (2017) Reference ranges for serum insulin-like growth factor I (IGF-I) in healthy Chinese adults. *PLoS One* 12(10): e0185561.

# CHAPTER 3

# Biochemical Parameters and Childhood Obesity

## INTRODUCTION

Childhood obesity is a multifaceted health concern for children and adolescents. It is considered when the weight of a child is above the normal weight for age and weight for height of their age group. It is largely influenced by multiple factors including heredity factors such as a person's behavior and genetics.

Childhood obesity can be defined as the excessive fat in the body that invariably affects the health of a child. Moreover, a generalized statement related to the excess fat for declaring obesity in the adolescents and children is lacking in the literature.

The study by Williams et al. (1992) of children (n=3,320) in the age range 5–18 years declared a classification for obesity. According to the authors, male participants were declared obese depending on the percentage of body fat up to 25%, while the female participants were classified as obese depending on the percentage of body fat up to 30% (Williams et al. 1992).

According to Flegal et al. (2002) and growth charts obtained from the Centers for Disease Control and Prevention in the United States, being overweight is defined as the nutritional status that is either up to or higher than the 95th percentile of the body mass index for age. Further, Flegal et al. (2002) defined nutritional status in-between the 85th to 95th percentile of the body mass index for age as "at-risk for overweight."

According to Ghosh (2014), scientists in European countries defined overweight as nutritional status up to or higher than the 85th percentile of the body mass index, while obesity as a condition up to or higher than the 95th percentile of the body mass index. Nawab et al. (2014) defined obesity as nutritional status either up to or greater than 95th percentile of the body mass index, whereas overweight was either up to or greater than the 85th percentile but less than the 95th percentile of body mass index.

## EPIDEMIOLOGY OF CHILDHOOD OBESITY

Prevalence of childhood obesity has increased throughout the world during the last decade. According to the International Obesity Task Force (2019), it was estimated that around 200 million children of school age were either obese or overweight.

According to Ogden et al. (2010), the proportion of obese children in the United States in 1980 was 7% in the age group 6–11 years. This had increased to 20% by 2008.

According to Kumar and Kelly (2007), the emergence of obesity in children is a major nutritional disorder in countries including the United States. They posited that one child out of every three is suffering from either being overweight or obesity. Childhood obesity is linked to comorbidities such as diabetes mellitus, dyslipidemia, hypertension, and obstructive sleep apnea. The generalized cause of obesity in children is a positive calorie balance owing to the intake of excessive calories along with a hereditary predisposition to obesity and being overweight.

Childhood obesity is a major and serious issue in the United States. According to the Centers for Disease Control and Prevention (CDC 2019), for children and adolescents in the age group 2–19 years, nearly 13.7 million children suffered from obesity, which amounted to a prevalence of 18.7% obesity in children and adolescents. Further, it was asserted by the CDC (2019) that the prevalence of obesity in Hispanics (25.8%) and in non-Hispanic blacks (22.0%) was higher in comparison to the prevalence of obesity in non-Hispanic whites (14.1%).

## ROLE OF SERUM LIPID PROFILE IN DIAGNOSIS OF CHILDHOOD OBESITY

Childhood obesity is linked to relatively raised levels of lipid profile, and obese children should be tested for hypercholesterolemia.

Friedland et al. (2002) studied the lipid profile in the obese and non-obese children. They selected 89 children and adolescents who were obese and 53 children who were non-obese and were age- and gender-matched. The authors posited that the serum cholesterol and triglycerides levels would be higher in the obese children in comparison to the non-obese children. They further described that nearly 50% of the obese children developed elevated serum cholesterol levels (hypercholesterolemia), where serum cholesterol level was greater than 170 mg/100 mL. Moreover, the severity of obesity in the children was unrelated to hypercholesterolemia (Friedland et al. 2002).

According to Medline Plus (2019), for any person aged 19 years or younger, the recommended serum cholesterol levels are as shown in Table 3.1.

According to some authors, children and adolescents in the United States have comparatively increased serum cholesterol levels, and U.S. adults suffer from a higher prevalence of coronary

TABLE 3.1    Recommended serum cholesterol levels

| Type of Cholesterol | Healthy Level |
| --- | --- |
| Total cholesterol | Less than 170 mg/dL |
| Non-HDL | Less than 120 mg/dL |
| LDL (low-density lipoprotein) | Less than 100 mg/dL |
| HDL (high-density lipoprotein) | More than 45 mg/dL |

Source: Medline Plus (2019).

artery disease (American Academy of Pediatrics 1998; Knuiman et al. 1983; Abraham et al. 1978).

According to a report by the American Academy of Pediatrics (1998), children and adolescents in the United States inflicted with dyslipidemia, are characterized by high plasma total cholesterol level, raised serum LDL cholesterol, and decreased serum HDL cholesterol levels. The prevalence of early onset coronary atherosclerosis is high in children and adolescents in the United States.

According to several authors (American Academy of Pediatrics 1998; Moll et al. 1983), children and adolescents who suffer from dyslipidemia and early coronary atherosclerosis have a hereditary predisposition to coronary artery disease (CAD) in their families.

## ROLE OF SERUM C-REACTIVE PROTEIN IN OBESITY

The C-reactive protein is the biomarker for low-grade inflammation. Further, obesity and cardiovascular disorder and maturity onset diabetes mellitus are linked to low-grade inflammation (Garcia et al. 2010).

The C-reactive protein signifies the low-grade inflammation that is manifested in response to inflammation in the liver and activation of adipocyte-derived pro-inflammatory cytokines (Pepys and Hirschfield 2003).

Lau et al. (2005) and Pasceri et al. (2000) are uncertain about the role of C-reactive protein in the pathogenesis of obesity, cardiovascular disorder, and diabetes mellitus.

Obesity is associated with the inflammatory process owing to the secretion of pro-inflammatory cytokines called adipokines (the proteins for cell signaling secreted by adipose tissues) (Conde et al. 2011). There is upregulation of adipokines during obesity. The elevated secretion in turn stimulates the synthesis and secretion of tumor necrosis factor alpha and interleukin-6. Moreover, the increased level of interleukin-6 has been linked to activation of hepatocytes and initiation of synthesis of a low-grade inflammation marker in the body called C-reactive protein (Panesar et al. 1999).

Adipocytes constitute the major cells in the adipose tissues. These cells store energy in the form of fat. However, in obesity, excess fat storage results in the physiological and morphological changes in the adipocytes. These cells undergo hyperplasia and hypertrophy. The hyperplastic changes in the adipocytes increase the synthesis of tumor necrosis factor-alpha and interleukin-6. These pro-inflammatory proteins induce low-grade inflammation in the adipose tissues and in the systemic tissues (Kwon and Pessin 2013).

The C-reactive protein is synthesized in the hepatocytes under the regulation of interleukin-6 (Pepys and Hirschfield 2003; Ross 1999). The hepatocytes contribute to nearly a quarter of the total circulating interleukin-6 in the body.

The C-reactive protein is considered the non-specific biomarker of low-grade inflammation and the liver was considered the only organ that could synthesize the C-reactive protein. Recently, it has been confirmed that adipocytes serve as extrahepatic tissues for the synthesis of C-reactive protein. Interleukin-6 is implicated in the induction of C-reactive protein synthesis in the liver, while tumor necrosis factor-alpha is considered as the chief pro-inflammatory protein, which is secreted by adipose tissues and is involved in the inflammation in the adipose tissues and it, in turn, contributes to the synthesis of C-reactive protein (Danesh et al. 1999).

Visser et al. (2001) conducted a study to find out the correlation between overweight and low-grade inflammation in the children. In the study, a total of 3,512 children were selected. The authors considered increased serum C-reactive protein (CRP) levels as $CRP \geq 0.22$ mg per 100 mL. Visser et al. (2001) reported the prevalence of increased levels of C-reactive protein in the overweight children in comparison to the normal children.

## REFERENCES

Abraham, S., Johnson, C.L., and Carroll, M.D. (1978) *Total Serum Cholesterol Levels of Children 4–17 Years: United States, 1971–74.* Hyattsville, MD: U.S. Department of Health, Education, and Welfare.

American Academy of Pediatrics (1998) Cholesterol in childhood: Committee on Nutrition. *Pediatrics* 101(1): 141–147.

Centers for Disease Control and Prevention (2019) Childhood obesity facts: Prevalence of childhood obesity in the United States. Available at: www.cdc.gov/obesity/data/childhood.html

Chinkes, D.L. (2005) Methods for measuring tissue protein breakdown rate in vivo. *Current Opinion in Clinical Nutrition and Metabolic Care* 8(5): 534–537.

Conde, J., Scotece, M., Gómez, R., López, V., Gómez-Reino, J.J., Lago, F., and Gualillo, O. (2011) Adipokines: Biofactors from white adipose tissue. A complex hub among inflammation, metabolism, and immunity. *Biofactors* 37(6): 413–420.

Danesh, J., Muir, J., and Wong, Y.-K. (1999) Risk factors for coronary heart disease and acute-phase proteins: A population-based study. *European Heart Journal* 20: 954–959.

Flegal, K.M., Wei, R., and Ogden, C. (2002) Weight-for-stature compared with body mass index-for-age growth charts for the United States from the Centers for Disease Control and Prevention. *American Journal of Clinical Nutrition* 75: 761–766.

Friedland, O., Nemet, D., Gorodnitsky, N., Wolach, B., and Eliakim, A. (2002) Obesity and lipid profiles in children and adolescents. *Journal of Pediatric Endocrinology and Metabolism* 15(7): 1011–1016.

Garcia, C., Feve, B., and Ferré, P. (2010) Diabetes and inflammation: Fundamental aspects and clinical implications. *Diabetes & Metabolism* 36(5): 327–338.

Ghosh, A. (2014) Explaining overweight and obesity in children and adolescents of Asian Indian origin: The Calcutta childhood obesity study. *Indian Journal of Public Health* 58: 125–128.

International Obesity Task Force (2019) Available at: www.iaso.org/iotf

Isley, W.L., Underwood, L.E., and Clemmons, D.R (1983) Dietary components that regulate serum somatomedin-C concentrations in humans. *Journal of Clinical Investigation* 71: 175–182.

Knuiman, J.T., Westenbrink, S., and van der Heyden, L. (1983) Determinants of total and high density lipoprotein cholesterol in boys from Finland, the Netherlands, Italy, the Philippines and Ghana with special reference to diet. *Human Nutrition: Clinical Nutrition* 37: 237–254.

Kumar, S. and Kelly, A.S. (2007) Review of childhood obesity: From epidemiology, etiology, and comorbidities to clinical assessment and treatment. *Mayo Clinic Proceedings* 92(2): 251–265.

Kwon, H. and Pessin, J.E. (2013) Adipokines mediate inflammation and insulin resistance. *Frontiers in Endocrinology* 4: 71.

Lau, D.C., Dhillon, B., Yan, H., Szmitko, P.E., and Verma, S. (2005) Adipokines: Molecular links between obesity and atherosclerosis. *American Journal of Physiology: Heart and Circulatory Physiology* 288(5): 2031–2041.

Medline Plus: U.S. National Library of Medicine (2019) High cholesterol in children and teens. Available at: https://medlineplus.gov/highch olesterolinchildrenandteens.html

Moll, P.P., Sing, C.F., and Weidman, W.H. (1983) Total cholesterol and lipoproteins in school children: Prediction of coronary heart disease in adult relatives. *Circulation* 67: 127–134.

Nawab, T., Khan, Z., Khan, I.M., and Ansari, M.A. (2014) Influence of behavioral determinants on the prevalence of overweight and obesity among school going adolescents of Aligarh. *Indian Journal of Public Health* 58: 121–124.

Ogden, C.L., Carroll, M.D., Curtin, L.R., Lamb, M.M., and Flegal, K.M. (2010) Prevalence of high body mass index in US children and adolescents, 2007–2008. *JAMA* 303: 242–249.

Panesar, N., Tolman, K., and Mazuski, J.E. (1999) Endotoxin stimulates hepatocyte interleukin-6 production. *Journal of Surgical Research* 85(2): 251–258.

Pasceri, V., Willerson, J.T., and Yeh, E.T. (2000) Direct proinflammatory effect of C-reactive protein on human endothelial cells. *Circulation* 102(18): 2165–2168.

Pepys, M.B. and Hirschfield, G.M. (2003) C-reactive protein: A critical update. *Journal of Clinical Investigation* 111: 1805–1812.

Ross, R. (1999) Atherosclerosis: An inflammatory disease. *New England Journal of Medicine* 240: 115–126.

Takeda, H., Ishihama, K., Fukui, T., Fujishima, S., Orii, T., Nakazawa, Y., Shu, H.J., and Kawata, S (2003). Significance of rapid turnover proteins in protein-losing gastroenteropathy. *Hepato-Gastroenterology* 50: 1963–1965.

Visser, M., Bouter, L.M., McQuillan, G.M., Wener, M.H., and Harris, T.B. (2001) Low-grade systemic inflammation in overweight children. *Pediatrics* 107(1): E13.

Williams, D.P., Going, S.B., Lohman, T.G., Harsha, D.W., Srinivasan, S.R., and Webber, L.S. (1992) Body fatness and risk for elevated blood-pressure, total cholesterol, and serum-lipoprotein ratios in children and adolescents. *American Journal of Public Health* 82: 527.

World Health Organization (1999) *Management of Severe Malnutrition: A Handbook for Higher Level Health Professionals (Doctors, Nurses, Nutritionists and Others) and Their Auxiliary Teams.* Brasilia: World Health Organization.

# CHAPTER 4

# Biochemical Parameters and Childhood Nutritional Anemia

## INTRODUCTION

Childhood nutritional anemia is a major health problem throughout the world, with a global prevalence in children and pregnant and lactating women.

It is caused by a deficiency in micronutrients such as iron, vitamin B12, and folic acid in the diet. Additionally, the involvement of trace minerals, such as zinc, selenium, and copper has been considered in the pathogenesis of nutritional anemia in children. It has been substantiated that micronutrients are closely associated with the process of erythropoiesis in bone marrow (Gupta 2017).

Anemia is the clinical condition that refers to a decline in the level of hemoglobin lower than the reference value, which is determined in reference to the age and sex of the individual (WHO 2001a). Iron deficiency is a health hazard affecting around 2 billion people globally.

Stoltzfus and Dreyfuss (1998) reported high prevalence of iron deficiency anemia in children aged between the ages of six months and two years.

According to a report by de Benoist et al. (2008), in a survey from 1993 to 2005, the highest anemia prevalence (47.4%) was found in preschool children and the lowest anemia prevalence (12.7%) was reported in adult males.

Iron deficiency in children and infants affects the development of brain. The level of iron in the fetus is determined by iron concentration in the body of the mother, and disorders in pregnancy such as diabetes mellitus and hypertension. In pregnant women suffering from diabetes mellitus, the developing baby passes through phases of hypoxic hypoxia. As a compensatory mechanism, a process of erythropoiesis is activated that demands extra iron, which is diverted toward bone marrow. The infant after birth suffers from polycythemia and impaired brain development if the plasma iron level is deficient in the body of the infant (Georgieff et al. 1990).

Lozoff and Georgieff (2006) studied the influence of iron deficiency on the neurodevelopment of animal models. The authors posited impaired dendritic structure in the hippocampal lobe. Further, iron deficiency was involved in the metabolism of monoamine oxidase enzyme and the process of myelination in animal models.

The biosynthesis of hormones like dopamine and serotonin requires the presence of iron in adequate concentration in the brain tissues. Iron deficiency is associated with impaired secretion of hormones and the alteration in the functioning of these hormones, especially during periods of rapid growth in children. Pre-term infants suffer more acutely from iron deficiency.

Growth of the fetus, pre-term infants, low birth weight, and iron deficiency are interrelated. Iron deficiency anemia results in hypoxic hypoxia in the body of pregnant women, which in turn activates the juxtamedullary apparatus in the kidneys. Hormones like angiotensin, aldosterone, and adrenaline are released. All these factors together favor the pathogenesis of preeclampsia and have harmful effects on the growing fetus. It has been observed that the presence of a high concentration of cortisol in maternal circulation negatively affects the fetus (Gupta 2017).

Allen (2001) mentioned the correlation among the hemoglobin concentration of pregnant women, concentration of human placental lactogen, and concentration of human chorionic gonadotropin. Iron deficit and reduced hemoglobin concentration induce the release of these hormones in pregnant women.

Grantham-McGregor and Ani (2001) posited the harmful effects of iron deficiency anemia on the brain development of children. The authors described impaired motor skills and affected development of cognitive processes in those children.

Felt and Lozoff (1996) studied the effect of iron deficiency on brain development in rats. Iron is essential for the synthesis and release of hormones such as dopamine and serotonin in the brain tissues. Iron deficit condition results in the reduced secretion of these hormones. Additionally, reduced secretion of hormones results in hypomyelination.

Iron deficiency influences the behavior of children in the formative period. It affects the social behavior, cognitive development, and attention span of children (Lozoff et al. 1991).

Iron deficiency reduces the oxygen-carrying capacity of hemoglobin in children. It results in anemic hypoxia and reduced perfusion of blood to the vital organs of the body (Zhu and Haas 1999).

Anemic hypoxia decreases the performance of children due to poor muscle contractility, and children are fatigued. Furthermore, the poor and delayed motor development is due to anemic hypoxia and ischemia in the muscles (Harahap et al. 2000).

Iron deficiency and iron deficiency anemia reduce the activity of protein kinase C that in turn is essential for the proliferation of T-lymphocytes and cell mediated immunity in children (Kuvibidila et al. 1999). The authors studied the role of iron deficiency and its effect on the activity of protein kinase C in mice.

## HEMOGLOBIN ESTIMATION

*Hemoglobinometry* refers to estimation of the concentration of hemoglobin in the bodies of individuals. It involves various methods, and each method has its own principle, advantages, and disadvantages.

The Haldane method is based upon the assessment of the carbon monoxide-transporting ability of blood. It is one of the oldest methods of hemoglobin estimation. It requires a source of carbon monoxide for using as reference (Clegg and King 1942). It is not used in the laboratory for hemoglobin estimation, and has been superseded by better, more modern methods.

The Dare method comprises a chamber of glass in which the blood is filled through capillary action. The glass chamber is illuminated by an electric bulb. The color of the blood is compared with the reference that depicts the concentration of hemoglobin (Stone et al. 1984).

The Lovibond-Drabkin method of hemoglobin estimation makes use of the cyanmethemoglobin concentration in the blood. In this method, a solution is mixed with the sample of blood and is kept for three minutes. The hemoglobin concentration is estimated from the comparison of the color of blood with the disc containing a standard color. Van Lerberghe et al. (1983) posited the higher sensitivity of this method in comparison to the other method that makes use of a comparator. The cost of the disc is the limiting factor in the use of the Lovibond-Drabkin method.

The Tallquist method utilizes a small strip of blotting paper where a drop of blood is added. The color of blood is matched with the standard (Elwood and Jacob 1966).

### The Cyanmethemoglobin Method

The *direct* cyanmethemoglobin method makes use of the chemical reaction involving the change of hemoglobin into cyanmethemoglobin. The absorbance is read at 540 nm in the colorimeter (Nkrumah et al. 2011).

The color intensity is directly proportional to hemoglobin concentration. A solution of 5 mL Drabkin is mixed with the fixed quantity of blood. It is kept undisturbed for two to four hours. The intensity of color of cyanmethemoglobin is recorded at 540 nm in the colorimeter. The method is regarded as the gold standard for estimation of hemoglobin.

The method requires venipuncture to collect a blood sample. Additionally, technical staff, a laboratory setup, and medical personnel are required to perform the method. Therefore, its use in villages and remote locations is difficult. Shah et al. (2011) mentioned the use of the method in the laboratories in rural areas. Furthermore, the method has disadvantages. Initially, the toxicity of cyanide is a limiting factor. Second, turbidity in the method results in inaccuracy.

The *indirect* cyanmethemoglobin method is best suited for the areas with limited medical facility for the screening of anemia. The method uses 20 μL of sample of blood that is added over the Whatman No. 1 filter paper. The dried and stained filter paper is packed into a plastic bag. It is dipped into the test tube containing 5 mL of Drabkin solution. The blood spot and solution interact for five minutes and are kept undisturbed for two hours. The intensity of the color is recorded at 540 nm.

### HemoCue Method

HemoCue is the portable and rapid method of estimation of hemoglobin. It is comprised of a battery-based photometer and microcuvettes.

In the microcuvette, 10 μL of the blood sample is loaded. Blood is mixed with sodium deoxycholate. The red blood cells are hemolyzed and hemoglobin is mixed with sodium nitrite that in turn converts the hemoglobin into methemoglobin.

The reaction proceeds with the interaction of methemoglobin with the sodium azide that results in formation of azide-methemoglobin, whose absorbance is read at a wavelength of 565 nm and another wavelength of 880 nm. The HemoCue method can be completed in 40 to 60 seconds (Ingram and Lewis 2000). HemoCue is the quantitative method that is highly suitable for the screening of anemia in surveys. According to Akhtar et al. (2009), the method has a specificity of 95.2% and a sensitivity of 94.1% in comparison to the direct cyanmethemoglobin method's specificity of 90.1% with a sensitivity of 94.2%.

Dacie and Lewis (2001) confirmed the utility of the HemoCue method in the multipurpose field surveys of the health of children.

## Sahli's Method

This method is a laboratory-based method of hemoglobin estimation. It requires a sample of blood in a hemoglobin test tube. Blood sample is mixed with 0.1 N HCl. The hemoglobin is converted into a dark brown hematinic acid. The intensity of the color is matched with the standard provided inside the Sahli's hemoglobinimeter.

It is an easy, rapid, and economical method of hemoglobin estimation. However, there is subjective error in the color matching with the standard, and the sensitivity and specificity of the method is lower than the cyanmethemoglobin method in assessing anemia in field surveys (Balasubramaniam and Malathi 1992).

Sahli's method is used in primary health centers (PHCs) and hospitals (Barduagni et al. 2003) for the estimation of hemoglobin. However, it is subject to bias in the comparison of color with the standard. Moreover, the cyanmethemoglobin method is more sensitive than the Sahli method as far as its use in hospitals is concerned (Balasubramaniam and Malathi 1992).

## Automated Hematology Analyzer

The automated hematology analyzer is the most accurate but costly method of hemoglobin estimation. The method requires trained staff and laboratory facility. It is unsuited for the field surveys. It has a higher precision level in comparison to the HemoCue method.

## NBM-200

The NBM-200 method is comprised of a sensor and is the non-invasive method of hemoglobin estimation. The sensor is placed on the thumb and a digital reading is recorded (Kim et al. 2013). The NBM-200 is equipped with lesser sensitivity and specificity than the HemoCue method (Kim et al. 2013).

## World Health Organization Color Scale Method

The WHO color scale method is a cheap, rapid, and easy method of hemoglobin estimation. It is best suited in field studies for the screening of anemia in children and pregnant women, where medical facilities and laboratory apparatus are limited.

The color scale is comprised of six shades of red representing the hemoglobin concentration. The values attributed to the shades are 4 g, 6 g, 8 g, 10 g, 12 g, and 14 g per 100 mL (WHO 2001b).

The six shades are placed over the polyvinyl chloride sheet. In the procedure, a blood drop is mounted over filter paper that appears as a spot. The color of the blood spot is matched with the standard.

This method is employed in epidemiological surveys, hospitals, and pediatric wards to estimate anemia.

The color scale method is a semi-qualitative method for estimation of hemoglobin. Its success is high in remote areas with inadequate laboratory facilities. In rural areas, the color scale method is a laboratory procedure and according to the WHO (2001b), the method has 95% sensitivity and 99.5% specificity.

The color scale method can be used for the detection of hemoglobin among infants of four months old (van Rheenen and de Moor 2007). In another study by Montresor et al. (2000), the color scale method is appropriate for use in surveys. Darshana and Uluwaduge (2014) confirmed the utility of the color scale method in screening for anemia during the blood donation camps. Furthermore, color scale reading is subject to variation if it is used by different technicians for the same patient.

## Transferrin Saturation Test

Transferrin saturation is the ratio between serum iron concentration and the total iron binding capacity of transferrin. It is presented as a percentage. Its reference value lies between 20% and 50%. It signifies the saturation ability of transferrin. Transferrin saturation level below 20% is indicative of a deficiency of iron in the body. The normal value of transferrin saturation is between 15% and 50% in males, and between 12% and 45% in females (Camaschella 2015).

The transferrin is a globular protein. It is essential for the transport of iron molecules in the plasma. Each molecule of transferrin attaches to two molecules of iron. It transports the iron across the body tissues and delivers it to tissues. In the state of iron deficiency, the quantity of transferrin in the plasma is raised, whereas its concentration is reduced during hypoproteinemia in the body.

Huebers et al. (1987) proved that transferrin saturation below 15% is inadequate for the normal process of erythropoiesis daily. There would be iron deficiency erythropoiesis and the erythrocytes and reticulocytes would be affected in their shape and size.

The plasma transferrin concentration can be evaluated by immunological methods such as enzyme-linked immunosorbent assays (the technique using plates for detection of proteins, hormones, peptides, and antibodies). The immunoblotting assay (the proteins undergo denaturation and then denatured proteins pass through gel electrophoresis) utilizes either monoclonal or polyclonal antibodies. These methods have high sensitivity in the detection of plasma transferrin saturation (Huebers et al. 1987). These methods are better than the colorimetric method and atomic absorption spectrophotometry method. These methods are marked with limitations. There is variation in the affinity of antibodies to the epitopes on the transferrin. There is no internationally accepted standard for the comparison of different assays. These limitations could be a source of error in the determination of plasma transferrin concentration.

## Serum Iron/Total Iron Binding Capacity (TIBC)

This biochemical test for serum iron estimates the concentration of iron that circulates in the blood circulation. It remains attached to transferrin molecules in the plasma that sustains its mobility.

Around 65% of the total body iron exists in the conjugated form with globin in the hemoglobin and it is stored in the erythrocytes. Further, around 4% of the iron in body exists in the form of myoglobin in skeletal muscles.

The remaining 30% of the body iron is distributed in the liver, spleen, and bone marrow, and it is stored in these tissues in the form of hemosiderin and ferritin. Serum iron tests measure the circulating iron in the blood circulation and it is unable to detect the iron that is stored in the tissues.

The normal value of serum iron in males is 65–176 μg per 100 mL, in females its value is 50–170 μg per 100 mL, in newborn babies its value is 100–250 μg per 100 mL, and its value for children is 50–120 μg per 100 mL (Bunn 2015; Little et al. 2013). In children, iron deficiency is marked by a value of serum iron below 50 μg/100 mL.

The serum iron concentration is variable during the daytime. This diurnal variation becomes a limiting factor in its utility to detect iron deficiency anemia in population surveys.

## Serum Ferritin

The biochemical test for serum ferritin is indicative of total iron stores of the body. This test has an advantage over the hemoglobin test in that the former is independent of the altitude.

A fall in serum ferritin levels reflects the iron deficiency in the body in the absence of infection or inflammation in the body tissues.

The serum ferritin test is an important parameter for the iron stores of the body. The ferritin is an acute-phase response protein. The concentration of ferritin increases in the infection or inflammation. Therefore, it is not a true indicator of iron stores in the body during infection or inflammation.

Moreover, normal serum ferritin shows the iron stores in the body in the absence of infection or inflammation. Nevertheless, the serum ferritin test cannot be employed for the detection of iron deficiency anemia in population surveys in areas afflicted with a high occurrence of helminthes infection, malaria, and environmental enteropathy in children (Gupta 2017).

The normal reference range for males is 20–500 ng per 100 mL, whereas in females, it is 20–200 ng per 100 mL (Mayo Clinic 2019). In children (≥ 5 years), its value is 15 ng per 100 mL, and for children above 12 years of age, its value is 12 ng per 100 mL (WHO 2001a).

A value of serum ferritin below the reference value is indicative of low body iron stores, whereas a value higher than the reference value is marked by hemochromatosis, porphyria, hyperthyroidism, or leukemia (Mayo Clinic 2019).

## Serum Homocysteine Level

A biochemical test for homocysteine estimates the concentration of homocysteine in plasma. Homocysteine is a non-proteinogenic amino acid. It is a homolog of cysteine amino acid, with the difference being the presence of an additional methylene bridge. It is synthesized from methionine through the elimination of the terminal methyl group.

Homocysteine can be remethylated into methionine with the help of cobalamin. The reference value of serum homocysteine in adult males in Western populations is 10–12 μmol per liter and values close to 20 μmol/L are seen in older patients and populations with decreased serum vitamin B (Bots et al. 1999; Selhub et al. 2000).

Elevated levels of homocysteine in the plasma raise the probability of injury to the endothelial layer in blood vessels. Hyperhomocysteinemia could lead to inflammation in blood vessels. It could be a factor for atherogenesis and ischemic heart disease (Selhub 1999).

Mahmoud et al. (2014) studied the homocysteine levels and vitamin B12 concentrations in females suffering from iron deficiency anemia from the Gaza Strip. Blood samples were taken from 240 female students in the age range of 18–22 years for assessing parameters such as serum ferritin, blood count, vitamin B12, and homocysteine. Mahmoud et al. (2014) described that 20.4% of the female students had iron deficiency anemia. The authors confirmed a reduced serum vitamin B12 level (212.9 ± 62.8 pg per mL) in female students suffering from iron deficiency anemia in comparison to healthy controls (286.9 ± 57.1 pg per mL). Mahmoud et al. (2014) also described elevated serum homocysteine levels in the female students with iron deficiency anemia (27.0 ± 4.6 μmol per L) in comparison to healthy controls (15.5 ± 2.9 μmol per L).

A reciprocal and strong correlation between homocysteine levels and iron deficiency anemia in female students was confirmed, and the authors concluded that the serum homocysteine level is a biomarker for iron deficiency (Mahmoud et al. 2014).

## Serum Methylmalonic Acid

Cobalamin is a water-soluble vitamin. It plays a major functional role in the maintenance of nerve sheaths and erythropoiesis. The deficiency of cobalamin in the body is associated with pernicious anemia and neurological manifestations like peripheral neuropathy, paresthesia, and demyelination of the corticospinal tract (Oh and Brown 2003; Schloss et al. 2015).

The deficiency of vitamin B12 can result from malabsorption syndrome, dietary deficiency or carcinoma of gastric mucosa. Chronic alcoholism and old age are predisposing factors to vitamin B12 deficiency (Allen 2009).

Methylmalonic acid is converted into methyl malonyl-CoA and ultimately into succinyl-CoA with the help of vitamin B12 as cofactor. Deficiency of vitamin B12 can lead to a rise in serum methylmalonic acid that becomes the biomarker of vitamin B12 deficiency and associated nutritional anemia in children.

Savage et al. (1994) conducted a study comprising 406 patients suffering from deficiency of vitamin B12. The authors described a 98.4% sensitivity of serum methylmalonic acid.

Lindenbaum et al. (1990) conducted a study on patients with pernicious anemia. The authors confirmed a rise in the serum levels of methylmalonic acid and homocysteine in the patients before the decline in serum vitamin B12 levels.

The estimation of serum vitamin B12 is necessary in pernicious anemia. This test confirms the low level of cobalamin in patients with anemia. Allen et al. (1990) confirmed that low cobalamin serum levels could not be associated with a deficiency of cobalamin. Therefore, it is necessary to perform an additional test to confirm the cobalamin-deficient patients. The serum methylmalonic acid level rises in vitamin B12 deficiency and its level is normalized after the treatment of the patient with cobalamin supplements.

## Intrinsic Factor Antibody Test

Intrinsic factor is a glycoprotein that is related to the cobalamin transport proteins family. It is secreted by the parietal cells of the gastric mucosa. It is essential for the absorption of vitamin B12 in the intestine. Vitamin B12 binds with the intrinsic factor through the receptor-mediated endocytosis in the mucosa of ileum and forms vitamin B12 1/n intrinsic factor complex. It enters the hepatic portal circulation (NHS 2019).

Pernicious anemia is the outcome of the autoimmune disorder that affects the gastric mucosa. The parietal cells are damaged and the secretion of intrinsic factors is decreased. Furthermore, the auto-antibodies to intrinsic factors interfere in the binding of vitamin B12 to intrinsic factor by blocking the sites (NHS 2019).

The intrinsic factor antibodies are of two types: intrinsic factor blocking antibodies that interfere with the binding of vitamin B12 on the binding sites of the intrinsic factor and intrinsic factor binding antibodies that attach to various sites on the intrinsic factor, resulting in the inhibition of binding of intrinsic factor–vitamin B12 complex to binding sites in the small intestine (NHS 2019).

The detection of intrinsic factor antibodies and a decline in vitamin B12 levels are diagnostic of pernicious anemia.

According to the NHS (2019), a value less than 1.20 AU/mL is considered negative for the screening of the intrinsic factor antibody. Further, a value between 1.21 and 1.52 AU/mL is considered borderline (NHS 2019). According to the NHS (2019), a value higher than 1.53 AU/mL is labeled as positive for the intrinsic factor antibody.

Khan et al. (2009) hypothesized that intrinsic factor antibodies could be detected in around 70% of patients with vitamin B12 deficiency. The authors conducted a study to examine the correlation between vitamin B12 level and intrinsic factor antibodies. They found that only four patients (0.47%) had intrinsic factor antibodies present with low vitamin B12 and confirmed that the intrinsic factor antibody test is confirmation for pernicious anemia. But its level is not related to vitamin B12 levels (Khan et al. 2009).

## Serum Folate Test

Serum folate is found in the form of N-(5)-methyl tetrahydrofolate. The folate is partly absorbed in the small intestine from dietary sources and it is partly synthesized by the colonic microbes (Benoist 2008; George et al. 2002).

As dietary folate consumption is reduced, serum folate levels decline after a few days, whereas, the erythrocyte-folate levels are not subject to variation on the basis of dietary fluctuations (Benoist 2008; George et al. 2002).

The deficiency of folate is linked with megaloblastic anemia and macrocytosis. Folate deficiency is reported commonly in pregnant women, alcoholics, and those suffering from malnutrition.

According to Benoist (2008) and George et al. (2002), a reference value equal to or greater than 4.0 µg/L is considered a normal folate level, whereas a value less than 4.0 µg/L is labeled as a folate deficiency.

Kapil et al. (2015) hypothesized that a deficiency of folate and cobalamin interplay in nutritional anemia in children in the age group of 12–59 months. The authors conducted a cross-sectional study that was comprised of 470 children. Venous blood samples were taken and dietary patterns were studied by the authors (Kapil et al. 2015). They detected an overall prevalence of deficiency in cobalamin (180 out of 469, 38.4%) and a deficiency of folate (263 out of 416, 63.2%) in children. Kapil et al. (2015) concluded a high prevalence of deficiency in cobalamin and folate in children below five years of age.

## REFERENCES

Akhtar, K., Sherwani, R.K., Rahman, L., et al. (2000) HemoCue photometer: A better alternative of hemoglobin estimation in blood donors? *Indian Journal of Hemotology and Blood Transfusion* 24: 170–172.

Allen, L.H. (2001) Biological mechanisms that might underlie iron's effect on foetal growth and preterm birth. *Journal of Nutrition* 131: S581–S589.

Allen, L.H. (2009) How common is vitamin B-12 deficiency? *American Journal of Clinical Nutrition* 89(2): S693–S696.

Allen, R.H., Stabler, S.P., Savage, D.G., and Lindenbaum, J. (1990) Diagnosis of cobalamin deficiency I: Usefulness of serum methylmalonic acid and total homocysteine concentrations. *American Journal of Hematology* 34(2): 90–98.

Balasubramaniam, P. and Malathi, A. (1992) Comparative study of hemoglobin estimated by Drabkin's and Sahli's methods. *Journal of Postgraduate Medicine* 38: 8–9.

Barduagni, P., Ahmed A.S., Curtale, F., Raafat, M., and Soliman, L. (2003) Performance of Sahli and colour scale methods in diagnosing anaemia among school children in low prevalence areas. *Tropical Medicine & International Health* 8: 615–618.

Benoist, B.D. (2008) Conclusions of a WHO Technical Consultation on folate and vitamin B12 deficiencies. *Food and Nutrition Bulletin* 29(2): S238–S244.

Bots, M.L., Launer, L.J., Lindemans, J., Hoes, A.W., Hofman, A., Witteman, J.C.M., Koudstaal, P.J., and Grobbee, D.E. (1999) Homocysteine and short-term risk of myocardial infarction and stroke in the elderly. *Archives of Internal Medicine* 159(1): 38–44.

Bunn, H.F. (2015) Approach to the anemias. In L. Goldman and A.I. Schafer (eds.), *Goldman-Cecil Medicine*, 25th ed. Philadelphia, PA: Elsevier Saunders.

Camaschella, C. (2015) Iron-deficiency anemia. *New England Journal of Medicine* 327(19): 1832–1843.

Clegg, J.W. and King, E.J. (1942) Estimation of haemoglobin by the Alkaline Haematin Method. *BMJ* 2: 329–333.

Dacie, J.V. and Lewis, S.M. (2001) *Practical Hematology*. Edinburgh: Churchill Livingstone.

Darshana, L.G. and Uluwaduge, D.I. (2014) Validation of the WHO Hemoglobin Color Scale Method. *Anemia*. Available at: www.ncbi. nlm.nih.gov/pubmed/24839555

de Benoist, B., McLean, E., Egli, I., and Cogswell, M. (eds.) (2008) *Worldwide Prevalence of Anaemia 1993–2005*. Geneva: World Health Organization.

Elwood, P.C. and Jacobs, A. (1966) Haemoglobin estimation: A comparison of different techniques. *BMJ* 1: 20–24.

Felt, B.T. and Lozoff, B. (1996) Brain iron and behaviour of rats are not normalized by treatment of iron deficiency anemia during early development. *Journal of Nutrition* 126: 693–701.

George, L., Mills, J.L., and Johansson, A.L. (2002) Plasma folate levels and risk of spontaneous abortion. *JAMA* 16(288): 1867–1873.

Georgieff, M.K., Landon, M.B., Mills, M.M., Hedlund, B.E., Faassen, A.E., Schmidt, R.L., Ophoven, J.J., and Widness, J.A. (1990) Abnormal iron distribution in infants of diabetic mothers: Spectrum and maternal antecedents. *Journal of Pediatrics* 117: 455–461.

Grantham-McGregor, S., and Ani, C. (2001) A review of studies on the effect of iron deficiency on cognitive development in children. *Journal of Nutrition* 131: S649–S668.

Gupta, A. (2017) *Nutritional Anemia in Preschool Children*. Singapore: Springer.

Harahap, H., Jahari, A.B., Husaini, M.A., Saco-Pollitt, C., and Pollitt, E. (2000) Effects of an energy and micronutrient supplement on iron deficiency anemia, physical activity, and motor and mental development in undernourished children in Indonesia. *European Journal of Clinical Nutrition* 54: S114–S119.

Huebers, H.A., Eng, M.J., Josephson, B.M., Ekpoom, N., Rettmer, R.L., Labbe, R.F., Pootrakul, P., and Finch, C.A. (1987) Plasma iron and transferrin iron-binding capacity evaluated by colorimetric and immunoprecipitation methods. *Clinical Chemistry* 33: 273–277.

Ingram, C.F. and Lewis, S.M. (2000) Clinical use of WHO haemoglobin colour scale: Validation and critique. *Journal of Clinical Pathology* 53: 933–937.

Kapil, U., Toteja, G.S., and Bhadoria, A.S. (2015) Cobalamin and folate deficiencies among children in the age group of 12–59 months in India. *Biomedical Journal* 38(2): 162–166.

Khan, S., Del-Duca, C., Fenton, E., Holding, S., Hirst, J., Doré, P.C., and Sewell, W.A. (2009) Limited value of testing for intrinsic factor antibodies with negative gastric parietal cell antibodies in pernicious anaemia. *Journal of Clinical Pathology* 62(5): 439–441.

Kim, M.J., Park, Q., Kim, M.H., Shin, J.W., and Kim, H.O. (2013) Comparison of the accuracy of noninvasive hemoglobin sensor (NBM-200) and portable hemoglobinometer (HemoCue) with an automated hematology analyzer (LH500) in blood donor screening. *Annals of Laboratory Medicine* 33: 261–267.

Kuvibidila, S.R., Kitchens, D., and Baliga, B.S. (1999) In vivo and in vitro iron deficiency reduces protein kinase C activity and translocation in murine splenic and purified T cells. *Journal of Cellular Biochemistry* 74: 468–478.

Lindenbaum, J., Savage, D.G., Stabler, S.P., and Allen, R.H. (1990) Diagnosis of cobalamin deficiency: II. Relative sensitivities of serum cobalamin, methylmalonic acid, and total homocysteine concentrations. *American Journal of Hematology* 34: 99–107.

Little, J.A., Benz, E.J., and Gardner, L.B. (2013) Anemia of chronic diseases. In R. Hoffman, E.J. Benz Jr. and L.E. Silberstein (eds.), *Hematology: Basic Principles and Practice*, 6th ed. Philadelphia, PA: Elsevier Saunders.

Lozoff, B. and Georgieff, M.K. (2006) Iron deficiency and brain development. *Seminars in Pediatric Neurology* 13: 158–165.

Lozoff, B., Jimenez, E., and Wolf, A.W. (1991) Long-term developmental outcome of infants with iron deficiency. *New England Journal of Medicine* 325: 687–694.

Mayo Clinic (2019) Ferritin test. Available at: www.mayoclinic.org/tests-procedures/ferritin-test/about/pac-20384928

Montresor, A., Albonico, M., Khalfan, N., Stoltzfus, R.J., Tielsch, J.M., Chwaya, H.M., and Savioli, L. (2000) Field trial of a haemoglobin colour scale: An effective tool to detect anaemia in preschool children. *Tropical Medicine and International Health* 5: 129–133.

NHS Foundation Trust (2019) Intrinsic factor antibodies. Available at: www.southtees.nhs.uk/services/pathology/tests/intrinsic-factor-antibodies/

Nkrumah, B., Nguah, S.B., Sarpong, N., Dekker, D., Idriss, A., May, J., and AduSarkodie, Y. (2011) Hemoglobin estimation by the HemoCue®

portable hemoglobin photometer in a resource poor setting. *BMC Clinical Pathology* 11: 5.

Oh, R. and Brown, D.L. (2003) Vitamin B12 deficiency. *American Family Physician* 67(5): 979–986.

Savage, D.G., Lindenbaum, J., Stabler, S.P., and Allen, R.H. (1994) Sensitivity of serum methylmalonic acid and total homocysteine determinations for diagnosing cobalamin and folate deficiencies. *American Journal of Medicine* 96: 239–246.

Schloss, J.M., Colosimo, M., Airey, C., and Vitetta, L. (2015) Chemotherapy-induced peripheral neuropathy (CIPN) and vitamin B12 deficiency. *Supportive Care in Cancer* 23(7): 1843–1850.

Selhub, J. (1999) Homocysteine metabolism. *Annual Review of Nutrition* 19: 217–246.

Selhub, J., Jacques, P.F., Bostom, A.G., Wilson, P.W., and Rosenberg, I.H. (2000) Relationship between plasma homocysteine and vitamin status in the Framingham study population: Impact of folic acid fortification. *Public Health Reviews* 28(1–4): 117–145.

Shah, V.B., Shah, B.S., and Puranik, G.V. (2011) Evaluation of non-cyanide methods for hemoglobin estimation. *Indian Journal of Pathology and Microbiology* 54: 764–768.

Sirdah, M.M., Yassin, M.M., El Shekhi, S, and Lubbad, A.M. (2014) Homocysteine and vitamin B12 status and iron deficiency anemia in female university students from Gaza Strip, Palestine. *Revista Brasileira de Hematologia e Hemoterapia* 36(3): 208–212.

Stoltzfus, R.J. and Dreyfuss, M.L. (1998) *Guidelines for the Use of Iron Supplements to Prevent and Treat Iron Deficiency Anaemia.* Geneva: INACG/WHO/UNICEF.

Stone, J.E., Simmons, W.K., Jutsum, P.J., and Gurney, J.M. (1984) An evaluation of methods of screening for anaemia. *Bulletin of the World Health Organization* 62: 115–120.

van Lerberghe, W., Keegels, G., Cornelis, G., Ancona, C., Mangelschots, E., and van Balen, H. (1983) Haemoglobin measurement: The reliability of some simple techniques for use in a primary health care setting. *Bulletin of the World Health Organization* 61: 957–965.

van Rheenen, P.F. and de Moor, L.T. (2007) Diagnostic accuracy of the haemoglobin colour scale in neonates and young infants in resource-poor countries. *Tropical Doctor* 37: 158–161.

World Health Organization (2001a) *Iron Deficiency Anaemia: Assessment, Prevention and Control: A Guide for Programme Managers.* Geneva: WHO.

World Health Organization (2001b) *Haemoglobin Color Scale: Practical Answer to a Vital Need.* Geneva: WHO.

Zhu, Y.I. and Haas, J.D. (1999) Altered metabolic response of iron depleted nonanemic women during a 15-km time trial. *Journal of Physiology* 84: 1768–1775.

# CHAPTER 5

# Biochemical Parameters: Childhood Diarrhea and Malabsorption Syndrome

## INTRODUCTION: CHILDHOOD DIARRHEA

Childhood diarrhea is a clinical condition manifested as passage of watery stools three times or more a day. Acute diarrhea is of short duration and persists generally for two to three days. Passage of stools of normal consistency more than normal frequency is not considered as diarrhea. Chronic diarrhea in children lasts for three to four weeks (NIDDK 2014).

Further, passing of loose stools in breastfed infants is not labeled as diarrhea (NDDI 2013). Generally, children below three years of age are affected by frequent episodes of diarrhea in developing countries (WHO 2013).

Diarrhea deteriorates the nutritional status of children. According to WHO (2013), diarrhea is the main cause of mortality in children under five years of age.

Chronic diarrhea is caused by gastrointestinal infection of bacteria like *Escherichia coli*, *Salmonella*, *Shigella*, and paratyphoid. The source of infection in diarrhea is the feco-oral route (Jill et al. 2010). The rotavirus is a highly contagious retrovirus (double stranded) that causes diarrhea in infants and children (Mayo Foundation 2019b). It has a high mortality rate in children causing about 215,000 deaths per annum in children. The infections result in difficulty in the digestion of carbohydrates or protein in some children. The duration of diarrhea is unnecessarily prolonged in children. The parasitic infections that cause diarrhea always require intensive therapy to eradicate the parasitic infection and cure diarrhea in children (NIDDK 2014).

Chronic diarrhea is also caused by food allergy, lactose intolerance, inflammatory bowel disease, functional GIT disorders, celiac disease, and ulcerative colitis in children. Diarrhea decreases the immune status of affected children. It is the cause of child mortality for 1.5 million to 5 million children annually below the age of five (Bern et al. 1992). Diarrhea dehydrates the body tissues and drains minerals in children (UNICEF/WHO 2010).

Children in developing countries suffer from chronic diarrhea that persists for more than 14 days, also known as persistent diarrhea. Poor sanitization and contaminated drinking water are common causative factors in diarrhea in children in developing countries. Children also suffer from frequent attacks of chronic diarrhea.

## TODDLER'S DIARRHEA

Toddler's diarrhea in children is also called functional diarrhea and childhood chronic non-specific diarrhea. Toddler's diarrhea is a common chronic diarrhea in infants and toddlers (from six months) and children of preschool age (three years).

It is manifested as passing three or more watery loose stools per day. The children are free of any other types of symptoms. Further, these children have a normal pattern of growth. They have normal weight and height. Generally, the intake of a carbohydrate-rich diet in the age group is the cause of toddler's diarrhea. This diarrhea requires no treatment and is cured by the time children reach school age (NIDDK 2014).

## IRRITABLE BOWEL SYNDROME

Irritable bowel syndrome (IBS) is an additional common cause of chronic diarrhea in children. It is manifested as abdominal discomfort, cramps, gas, and bloating in the abdomen followed by episodes of constipation and diarrhea. A frequent change in bowel habits is the common symptom of this disorder.

The most common cause of IBS is behavioral changes in the children, such as anxiety, emotional disturbance, and depression. The age predilection of IBS is school-age children and adolescents. Food allergies and stress could trigger the symptoms of IBS.

## FOOD ALLERGY

A food allergy is the immunological response of the body to particular foods that are consumed. The common manifestations of food allergy are itching on skin, redness and swelling in the mouth, vomiting, diarrhea, difficulty in breathing, and a fall in blood pressure (U.S. National Library of Medicine 2019).

Food allergy manifests in the infancy stage (NIDDK 2014). Most children overcome the food allergy by the time they reach school age. According to Wood (2003), nearly 50% of infants overcome their food allergy by the end of the first year of life, and the remaining children resolve the allergy by the end of the fifth year.

Allergies to cow milk and soya protein are the most common food allergies in children (Gupta 2017). Others have allergy to cereals, eggs, and seafood. Allergy to cow milk protein manifests in the first year of life in 2–6% of infants (Host 2002).

Diarrhea and weight loss in children are the common manifestations of food allergy.

## CELIAC DISEASE

Celiac disease is an autoimmune disorder of the small intestine. It manifests in the genetically predisposed population of children and adults. Its prevalence is 1 in 100 persons in the world and an estimated 2.5 million Americans are affected by the disorder but are undiagnosed and could suffer serious outcomes from the disease (Celiac Disease Foundation 2019).

Gluten protein in wheat, barley, or rye triggers an immune response in the body. The immune response damages the villi in the small intestine. It decreases the absorption capability of the small intestine.

It can occur in any age group of children. It manifests as chronic diarrhea, gas, bloating, and abdominal cramps. The stools are pale colored and foul smelling (NIDDK 2014).

Malabsorption due to celiac disease in children thwarts the growth and development of children of preschool age. There is weight loss, failure of linear growth, anemia, and decreased serum calcium levels in children.

## LACTOSE INTOLERANCE

Lactose intolerance is a clinical condition characterized by a person's inability to digest lactose (milk sugar). It manifests as gas formation, bloating, cramps, and diarrhea after the intake of milk or milk products.

In general, lactose is the predominant milk sugar. It is digested in the alimentary canal by the lactase enzyme into glucose and galactose. These monosaccharides after digestion are absorbed into the blood circulation.

Owing to a deficiency of the lactase enzyme, the lactose is not digested completely in the small intestine. It is passed onto the large intestine as undigested foodstuff. It is called lactose malabsorption in children.

The undigested lactose is degraded by colonic bacteria. It produces gas and bloating. Lactase deficiency appears after the age of two years in children and it can manifest later in childhood during the adolescent period. Premature babies may develop lactose intolerance and diarrhea, but infants rarely suffer from lactose intolerance. Furthermore, hereditary lactase deficiency is a congenital condition that is rarely found in children (NIDDK 2014; Mayo Foundation 2019a).

## ULCERATIVE COLITIS

Ulcerative colitis is a clinical condition that is characterized by chronic inflammation of mucosa of the large intestine and formation of ulcers. The disease manifests as abdominal cramps, gas, diarrhea, mucus, bleeding, weight loss, and anemia in children.

The exact cause of ulcerative colitis is not known. It could be predisposed by the genetic constitution of person, lifestyle, stress, autoimmunity, and change in gut bacteria (NIDDK 2014). It is a type of inflammatory bowel disease. Studies have revealed that around 25% of cases exhibit manifestations in the adolescent age group (Abraham et al. 2012).

In children, the presence of chronic diarrhea (> 1 month duration) and recurrent episodes of diarrhea (more than two episodes in six months) is characteristic of ulcerative colitis (Abraham et al. 2012).

In a study by Abraham et al. (2012), a triad of symptoms of abdominal distress, chronic diarrhea, and loss of weight was seen in 25% of children while the other 25% of children reported abdominal distress, loss of appetite, and lethargy.

## IgA TISSUE TRANSGLUTAMINASE ANTIBODIES

Celiac disease is a chronic disorder affecting the small intestine and is in the group of inflammatory bowel disease.

It is caused by epitopes of the gluten protein in wheat, barley, and rye cereals. The disease manifests in genetically predisposed individuals and children.

The gluten peptides are taken up by antigen-presenting cells carrying HLA-DQ2- and HLA-DQ8 molecules and are presented efficiently to the helper T1 cell, in turn activating the T cytotoxic cell.

There is atrophy of villi in the small intestine and hyperplasia of crypts. The lamina propria and intra-epithelial regions are infiltrated with macrophages and inflammatory cells.

The tissue transglutaminase enzyme can stimulate the immuno-stimulatory effect of gluten through the process of deamidation. It also serves as target tissue antigen (autoantigen) to the immune system. The tissue transglutaminase enyme plays a significant role in the pathogenesis of celiac disease (Di Sabatino et al. 2012).

Tissue transglutaminase is a calcium cofactor dependent enzyme that catalyzes the post-translational modification of polypeptides. It results in the formation of an isopeptide bond between the γ-carboxamide group of glutaminyl residue and ε amino group of lysyl residue, which are present either in similar or different polypeptides (Folk and Finlayson 1977). Tissue transglutaminase enzyme is widely distributed in the body tissues. The tissue transglutaminase enzyme is concerned with the cross linking of peptides in the glutamine residue.

Tissue transglutaminase is involved in the regulation of cell homeostasis, apoptosis, and controlling cell cycles (Melino and Piacentini 1998).

IgA anti-tissue transglutaminase antibodies are considered useful in the detection of diarrhea caused by celiac disease. The test has high sensitivity and specificity.

Tissue transglutaminase enzyme reacts with the gluten pro-tein of cereals. There is formation of neoepitopes. These are the peptides which are attached to a class of major histocompatibility complex molecules. These constitute the antigenic determinants of neoantigens. These are fixed as a target for the T cells (Leclerc et al. 2019).

The immune response to these neoepitopes could initiate damage to the mucosa of the small intestine in celiac disease.

## IgA ENDOMYSIAL ANTIBODIES

The immunofluorescence or the enzyme-linked immunosor-bent assay techniques have been employed in the detection of circulating antibodies in celiac disease. These tests have varied sensitivity and specificity.

Chorzelski et al. (1983) mentioned the presence of a new antibody in primates that is produced against the membrane of smooth muscle bundles. The endomysium is the connective tissue that surrounds the smooth muscle bundles. It can take up silver stain. Recently, a target antigen in the endomysium was labeled as tissue transglutaminase (Dieterich et al. 1997).

Studies have demonstrated IgA endomysial antibodies and anti-tissue transglutaminase antibodies having sensitivity and specificity in more than 95% of celiac disease cases (Hill 2005).

## REFERENCES

Abraham, B.P., Mehta, S., and El-Serag, H.B. (2012) Natural history of pediatric-onset inflammatory bowel disease: A systematic review. *Journal of Clinical Gastroenterology* 46: 581–589.

Bern, C., Martines, J., De Zoyas, I., and Glass, R.L. (1992) The magnitude of the global burden of diarrhoeal disease. *PLoS One* 8(5): e64713.

Celiac Disease Foundation (2019) What is celiac disease? Available at: https://celiac.org/about-celiac-disease/what-is-celiac-disease/

Chorzelski, T.P., Sulej, J., Tchorzewski, H., Jablonska, S., Beutner, E.H., and Kumar, V. (1983) IgA class endomysium antibodies in dermatitis herpetiformis and coeliac disease. *Annals of the New York Academy of Sciences* 420: 325–334.

Dieterich, W., Ehnis, T., Bauer, M., Donner, P., Volta, U., Riecken, E.O., and Schuppan, D. (1997) Identification of tissue transglutaminase as the autoantigen of celiac disease. *Nature Medicine* 3(7): 797–801.

Di Sabatino, A., Vanoli, A., Giuffrida, P., Luinetti, O., Solcia, E., and Corazza, G.R. (2012) The function of tissue transglutaminase in celiac disease. *Autoimmunity Reviews* 11(10): 746–753.

Folk, J.E. and Finlayson, J.S. (1977) The ε-(γ-glutamyl)lysine cross-link and the catalytic role of transglutaminases. *Advances in Protein Chemistry* 31: 1–133.

Gupta, A. (2017) Nutritional anemia in preschool children. Available at: www.springer.com/gp/book/9789811051777

Hill, I.D. (2005) What are the sensitivity and specificity of serologic tests for celiac disease? Do sensitivity and specificity vary in different populations? *Gastroenterology* 128(4): S25–S32.

Host, A. (2002) Frequency of cow's milk allergy in childhood. *Annals of Allergy, Asthma & Immunology* 89(6): 33–37.

Jill, W.A., Wenjing, T., Lofgren, J., and Forsberg, B. (2010) Diarrhoeal diseases in low and middle income countries: Incidence, prevention and management. *Infectious Diseases Journal* 4(133): 113–124.

Leclerc, M., Mezquita, L., Guillebot De Nerville, G., Tihy, I., Malencia, I., Chouaib, S., and Mami-Chouaib, S. (2019) Recent advances in lung cancer immunotherapy: Input of T-cell epitopes associated with impaired peptide processing. *Frontiers in Immunology* 10: 1505.

Mayo Foundation for Medical Education and Research (2019a) Lactose intolerance. Available at: www.mayoclinic.org/diseases-conditions/lactose-intolerance/symptoms-causes/syc-20374232

Mayo Foundation for Medical Education and Research (2019b) Rotavirus. Available at: www.mayoclinic.org/diseases-conditions/rotavirus/symptoms-causes/syc-20351300

Melino, G. and Piacentini, M. (1998) Tissue transglutaminase in cell death: A downstream or a multifunctional upstream effector? *FEBS Letters* 430: 59–63.

National Digestive Diseases Information Clearing House (NDDI) (2013) Diarrhoea. Available at http://digestive.niddk.nih.gov/ddiseases/pubs/diarrhea

National Institute of Diabetes and Digestive and Kidney Diseases (NIDDK) (2014) Ulcerative colitis. Available at: www.niddk.nih.gov/health-information/digestive-diseases/ulcerative-colitis?dkrd=hispt0288

UNICEF/WHO (2010) Global, regional, and national causes of child mortality: An updated systematic analysis for 2010 with time trends since 2000. *Lancet* 380(9850): 1308.

U.S. National Library of Medicine (2019) Food allergy. Available at: https://medlineplus.gov/foodallergy.html

Wood, R.A. (2003) The natural history of food allergy. *Pediatrics* 111: 1631–1637.

World Health Organization (2013) Diarrhoeal disease. Available at www.who.int/news-room/fact-sheets/detail/diarrhoeal-disease

World Health Organization (2014) Available at: www.who.int/mediacentre/factsheets/fs330/en/

# Index

Printed in the United States
by Baker & Taylor Publisher Services